THE TRIATHLETE'S GUIDE TO
TRAINING WITH POWER

Dr. Philip Friere Skiba

PhysFarm Press

"Make everything as simple as possible, but not simpler."
- Albert Einstein -

Exercise can be beneficial for many people, but too much of anything can be dangerous to your health. This book describes cutting-edge training techniques used by extremely fit (often elite / professional / world-class) athletes. It is intended for educational purposes only. The techniques described herein are not a replacement for common sense, nor do they constitute medical advice. They should only be used after a complete and thorough examination by a trained physician. Your physician must agree that you are capable of performing heavy / maximal exercise for extended periods of time. If you have not been cleared for such exercise by your physician, you must not attempt anything you read here.

Philip Skiba and PhysFarm Training Systems LLC and LLP (UK) are not responsible for any conclusions drawn by the reader, nor any losses, injuries or illnesses that result directly or indirectly from attempting to use the techniques described herein. By reading this work and choosing of your own free will to apply any of the concepts, you specifically and completely accept and assume the risks inherent in undertaking any exercise training task or program, including illness, injury, disability and death, and the financial hardship that may result from any of those outcomes.

Copyright © 2008 by Philip Friere Skiba, D.O., M.S.

All rights reserved. Except for use in a review, reproduction or utilization of this work in any form or by any electronic, mechanical means, now known or hereafter invented is forbidden without the written permission of the author.

Printed in the United States of America.

ISBN: 978-0-9794636-1-7

Philip Friere Skiba
pskiba@physfarm.com
www.PhysFarm.com

Design and layout by Kathryn Skiba

Table of Contents

	Introduction	5
CHAPTER 1	You Want a Watt?	7
CHAPTER 2	Watt's Hard? Watt's Easy? Setting The Benchmark	13
CHAPTER 3	Plyometrics: Explosive Exercise To Develop Power	23
CHAPTER 4	Zones: The Specifics of Training	33
CHAPTER 5	Understanding Variability and Intensity	45
CHAPTER 6	How Much Are You Training? No, *really*.	53
CHAPTER 7	The Nuts and Bolts: Rationally Analyzing Your Training	59
CHAPTER 8	The Dose-Response View Of Training	71
CHAPTER 9	Intelligently Planning Your Training Season, Schedule, and Workout	83
CHAPTER 10	Guidelines For Racing	111
	Epilogue	115
	Works Cited	117
	About the Author	120

INTRODUCTION

To say I was pleasantly surprised at the success of my first book, *Scientific Training for Triathletes*, would be an understatement. It began as a grass roots effort to educate athletes about the function of their bodies. I figured I would sell a couple of copies to a few like-minded coaches, and that would be the end of it. Three years later, we have been through seven reprints, and sales of *Scientific Training for Triathletes* continue to increase every month! I like to think this is indicative of a collective hunger for trustworthy information about smart, healthy training.

Perhaps somewhat surprisingly, this isn't a textbook about bicycle power meters. Power-based training is a way of *thinking*, and not just something you do with a particular tool. It is a way of learning to think in terms of how much work you do, and how fast you do that work. This is important, because your body responds to those things very specifically. Once you understand the interplay of work and work rate, you will be able to analyze your past training and then plan future training with very specific results in mind.

That said, power training gets a lot easier when you have a few tools. Each of us has looked at a friend with a bicycle power measuring device and experienced some degree of "gear envy". The question is not, "Do I want one of those?" Of course you do. You also want, the shiny new GPS unit and that crazy looking stopwatch with twenty buttons on it. The real question is, "Will one of these devices make me train better and help me improve my performance?"

The answer to that question is a qualified yes. I say qualified because you must be willing to take the time to understand the data the power meter, GPS, or stopwatch is providing to you, and then be willing to act on that information in order to improve your training. If you aren't, save your money.

Much like *Scientific Training for Triathletes*, this book is about evidence-based training. What I mean by this is that there is no voodoo here. As much as is possible, everything I will relate to you is based upon published scientific research. Anything that represents my own educated opinion will be labelled as such. I do this because the scientific thought process informs my ideas, and I always want it to be clear where those ideas come from. I want you to have the opportunity to go back to the original sources of the data and evaluate it yourself. Do you believe it, or not? Do you think the authors made errors, or are they on top of their game? Sure, those guys are usually pretty smart, but so are you. Thinking critically will make you a better athlete or coach. Maybe you will come up with even better ideas!

It is my hope that *The Triathlete's Guide to Training with Power* will enable you to take your training and racing to the next level, and find that new elusive PR. At the end of the day, it is not about fancy supplements or fad training techniques. It is about hard work, using the best tools available, and rigorously applying the muscle between your ears. You can do it. This book is going to help.

CHAPTER 1
You Want a Watt?

The basic problem with power-based training is that most athletes (and a number of coaches) talk about "power" in the same way politicians talk about "values": they know people like the sound of it, but don't have the slightest idea of what it actually means.

With this in mind, let's begin with the basics: any exercise task requires you to do work. It takes work to pedal a bike to the end of the street, to walk up a flight of stairs, or to roll a keg of beer into a party. In the scientific world, work is measured in something called joules. A joule is equal to about 0.25 calories. It always takes the same number of joules to do the same work task. If your weight is constant, it always "costs" you the same number of joules to walk to the top of your stairs. However, you intuitively know that running up the stairs is somewhat harder than walking up the stairs. Why should this be? I just finished telling you that the same task (getting to the second floor) requires the same amount of work (joules), didn't I?

The difference is one of work *rate*. Running up the stairs requires you to do the same amount of work as walking up the stairs, but it requires that you do that work

> **Joule** - The measurement of work. Equal to about 0.25 calories.
>
> **Power** - Is an expression of work rate.
>
> **Watt** - The measurement of power. Equal to 1 joule per second.

much more quickly. Power is an expression of work rate. Running up the stairs requires more power, and that is why it feels harder. We measure power output in something called watts.

A watt is equal to 1 joule per second. That isn't particularly important, but we might as well get the definition out of the way so that we can move on to more pressing issues. The important point is this: to improve as an athlete, you need to be able to make more power. For instance, a slowpoke and an Olympian of identical body size can both run the mile, and it will cost each of them the same number of joules, more or less. The work task is identical. However, the Olympian gets to the finish line much more quickly because they are able to expend those joules more quickly. They are generating more watts.

As an athlete interested in improving, at the end of the day your goal is to be able to do the same. (In some cases, we could argue that the goal is to make the same number of watts over a longer period of time. However, it is usually pretty hard to do that without also giving yourself the ability to make more watts over a shorter period of time at some point.)

Making more watts sounds simple enough, however, there are many different ways to accomplish that goal. If you read my first book, *Scientific Training for Triathletes*, you realize that athletes exhibit very different, very specific responses to different types and amounts of training. Following wattage and associated markers will allow us to define and describe the particular types of training we are talking about. We should discuss why this is important. I mean, we talk about how we train all the time, even without power meters, right?

In simplistic terms, if I asked you how much training you did on the bike last week, how would you respond? It is a more difficult question than it might appear. If you responded by saying, "I put in about 100 miles," you really didn't tell me anything. You rode 100 miles, but you didn't say how fast you went. 100 miles at race pace is a lot harder than 100 miles of easy spinning with your friends.

Instead, you might say, "I put in about 100 miles at about 17 mph." Yet, even this statement does not tell the whole story. Is 17 mph fast for you? What percentage of your race pace does that translate into? Moreover, you really didn't **just** train at 17 mph, did you? You did a variety of different rides. Again, these details make important differences not only in communication, but also in your development as an athlete and your body's response to the training you do.

"Wait." You are about to tell me, "I wear a heart rate monitor. That tells me how hard I am going."

Er, sort of.

I'm going to break some bad news to you. Your heart rate is not a very good measure of training stress. The problem is that your heart rate is variable based not only on the exercise you are doing, but a lot of other stuff that has very little to do with the training task at hand. For instance, heat stress will make your heart rate higher at the same work rate. Overtraining may make it lower. Excitement will make it higher. Dehydration will make it higher. Lack of sleep plays a role. You get the idea here. Heart rate is just too unreliable. It's what we call a *dependent variable:* your heart rate is *dependent* upon all those things, *and* on how hard you exercise. You might **think** you are in Zone III (however you define that), but you might be in Zone II or IV. Or rather, your heart may in fact be in Zone III, but your legs are in Zone II or IV, and *your legs are what is most important.*

This doesn't mean that heart rate training doesn't work. It simply means the user has to be aware of all the caveats above in order to make best use of heart rate data. In contrast, the power meter removes all of this confusion.

Heart Rate Can Be Inflated By:
- Heat Stress
- Cardiac Drift
- Excitement
- Dehydration

It mechanically measures the work rate of your muscles. Your power output *always* accurately reflects your workout. For example, your 5-minute maximal power output is your 5-minute maximal power output, no matter how your heart responds to your attempt at generating it.

Now that we have an objective measurement of exercise intensity, we can both manage training and communicate about that training in terms everyone will understand. For instance, it doesn't matter that my 5-minute power is 300 watts, and yours is 400 watts. The point is that when either of us says that, we both understand what we mean and how intense that is. More importantly, training at that level will result in similar adaptations for the both of us: it will increase our VO2max, or our power output at VO2max, or both (among other things). We will discuss more of this in later chapters.

Knowing power output allows you to take things one step further. It allows you to objectively compare your abilities to others by expressing your power output per kilogram of your body weight. For instance, if you and I can both make 500 watts for 5 minutes, but you weigh 50 KG and I weigh 100 KG, you are clearly the better athlete. This is because *per kilogram of your body weight,* you are making 10 watts, whereas I am only making 5 watts. Thus, if we were climbing the same hill, you'd get to the top long before I would.

Interestingly, and as you might expect from some of the discussion above, we can also apply these concepts to running. In 2005, I invented the Gravity Ordered Velocity Stress Score (GOVSS) system. Without getting into a lot of painful math, it basically uses a combination of physics and physiology to calculate your power output for running.

Now, I'm sure you just raised your eyebrow and said, "Say what?" It's like this: for years runners trained on the basis of pace. This makes sense for the same reasons training with a power meter makes sense. However, it is just a little more complicated because pace is also dependent on the slope of the road you are running on.

What exactly is GOVSS?

As we've discussed in the book, the most important thing you can know about your workouts is your power output, because it tells you both how much work you did, and how fast you did it. That's great for cycling, because you can just buy a power meter. However, we can't do the same for running...can we?

As it turns out, you can actually calculate the power output of a runner utilizing a little math, and knowledge of the height and mass of the runner, their running speed, and the angle of the road. GPS directly measures all the needed variables, so it is sort of like a power meter for your body. Add the extra step of calculating the efficiency of the conversion of energy in the body to the outside world, and we're in business. This is what the GOVSS algorithm does. Although I devised it as a tool for sports scientists, it is now available to the public in Topofusion (http://www.topofusion.com) and in RaceDay (http://www.physfarm.com).

"Is this really necessary?" you may ask.

Think about this question for a moment: Is an 8-minute mile run on the flat just as hard as an 8-minute mile run up the side of a mountain? Of course not.

The difference between an 8-minute mile run on the flat and on a slope is one of power output. It takes more power to run the same speed going uphill, and you feel this by the sensation of increasing strain. GOVSS allows you to look at both efforts, and figure out how to equate the two. Now, it is possible to look at a hilly run, and figure out how fast you could have run on the flat, and vice versa. Now, we are getting somewhere...

GOVSS then goes one step further. It scores your workout on a points system, so you can directly compare workouts. It allows you to look at very different efforts and equate them in the sense of how much effect they had on you, metabolically speaking. For instance, you may do a tempo run of about 45 minutes, and a track workout of about 30 minutes, and you may wonder how they compare. If both gave you 50 GOVSS, you know the answer!

Running up a hill at 7 minutes per mile is a heck of a lot harder than running on the flat at 7 minutes per mile. Again, the difference is one of *power*. It takes more *power* to run up the hill at the same pace because you are fighting with gravity. The GOVSS system allows you to figure out just how much power different segments of different runs take, and then allows you to design your training program on that basis, rather than just kind of guessing about the impact of different kinds of hilly runs versus flat runs. We may think in terms of pace, because it is easy, but we *analyze* in terms of power to better understand what is going on with our training.

Finally, we can apply these concepts to swimming. Again, through some physics and physiology, we can actually make a pretty good calculation of how much power it takes to get through the water at particular speeds. This is important because it explains very nicely why it is easier to drop your time from 1:40 to 1:30 / 100M than it is to drop your time from 1:30 to 1:20. Both are a decrease of 10 seconds, but while you were increasing your speed linearly (by 10 seconds) the drag on your body (and thus the *power* required to increase speed) increased exponentially. This means not only that each increase in speed is harder, but that it is harder to make each increase than it was to make the previous increase. Again we, set up training zones in terms of speed, because that makes sense to us, but we can analyze the workout using *power* to better understand what it *meant*.

The point I am trying to drive home is this: it isn't just about how far or how fast you went. It is about understanding how much *work* you did, and how *fast* you did that work. Finally, we need to think about how much stress and strain the work / work rate put on your body, because your body responds according to the strain it endures. We'll discuss that just a bit later.

CHAPTER 2
Watt's Hard? Watt's Easy? Setting The Benchmark

Once you have purchased and installed the stopwatch / power meter / GPS of your choice, you need to get used to the thing. Don't plan on any major changes to your training program up front. Rather, spend a couple of weeks training as you normally would, then download the files. Look at your swimming logs in light of the actual recorded work and rest intervals. See how what you were actually doing compares to what you think you were doing. You'll likely be surprised.

Your first observation will most likely be that the numbers seem to jump around a lot. Your observation is correct. At any given instant, your power output or pace is varying substantially. What is important is that these seemingly arbitrary variations average out over time. This brings us to an important point: the human body responds according to averages. In other words, if you did a workout where you rode 10 seconds at 200 watts, then 10 seconds at 100 watts, and repeated this process for an hour, your body would respond (more or less) as though you'd just ridden that hour at 150 watts. The same goes for more standard workouts. The little variations in your intervals all average out in the end. You need to keep

> **The human body responds according to averages.**

CHAPTER 2
Watt's Hard? Watt's Easy? Setting the Benchmark

this in mind, and remember that while it is important to manage your power output in a broad sense, trying to manage it down to a couple of watts or less (i.e. the way you used to try to manage your heart rate) will likely drive you insane, and will probably not make much difference in the grand scheme of your training.

All this said, how do we determine what is hard and what is easy? How do we decide just how hard we have to train to improve in our races? I mean, it's nice to have all these numbers, but we need them to mean something to *us*. For the exercise intensities common in triathlon racing, an excellent way of doing this is by *relating an exercise task to our best power output for a one hour test or time trial*. You may have also heard this called "Functional Threshold Power (FTP). Of course, the problem with trying to relate training strain to a one hour test is that you need to go do a 1 hour test! There is an easier way to go about this, and it is by using something called Critical Power (CP), which we will explain shortly.

What is the rationale for the 1-hour power / Critical Power benchmarks? It is all about something called the Lactate Threshold (LT). You may have heard this term thrown around by your training buddies, or on Internet message boards. However, most people do not have a firm handle on what it means. Briefly, any time you exercise, you use both fat and carbohydrates for fuel. As you travel faster and faster, you switch your fuel mix to include relatively more carbohydrates, and relatively less fat. The by-product of burning that carbohydrate is lactate, which appears in your bloodstream. Thus, lactate makes a nice marker for exercise intensity. The point at which you make enough lactate to raise the blood level by 1 milimole is called LT (Figure 2-1). Very well trained athletes can go quite hard before they reach LT, whereas mere mortals like

> **Lactate Threshold (LT) -** A rise in serum lactate concentration of 1 milimole per liter over exercise baseline. Better athletes can generate more power / travel faster before this occurs.

myself reach it at more pedestrian paces. In fact, power output at LT is the best predictor of performance at race distances from just a few seconds out to stage races like the Tour de France!

Lactate is also nice for another reason: it exhibits a curvilinear pattern. In other words, it goes up from left to right kind of like a skateboard ramp; it gets steeper the harder you go. The reason why this is important is that LOTS of body processes exhibit a very similar looking curve. So, lactate tells us about our muscles, but the pattern also allows us to make some well-educated guesses about what is going on with our other body processes at the same time. We can therefore use it as a surrogate for overall physiologic stress. Later, we'll explain how we can weight our training using such a curve. As a rule of thumb, remember that stress rises with the 4th power of your power output in running or cycling, and about the 3rd power of your power output while swimming.

All this is well and good, however, most of us don't have lab testing gear out in the garage. How do we find this elusive LT? Fortunately, all you need is the power meter you just bought. You see, back in the 1980's, Dr. Ed Coyle figured out that LT is highly correlated with 1 hour maximal power.[1,2] Thus, you don't need to get a lot of blood drawn. Just fire up the power meter, head out on the bike, and kill yourself for an hour. Better yet, enter yourself in an ill-advised early season 40K TT, and see what kind of numbers you can put up. (In point of fact, a 1-hour TT done at a maximal pace

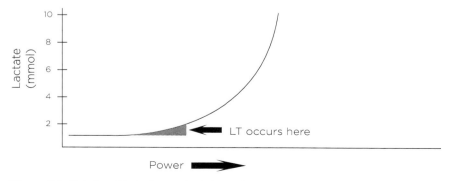

Figure 2-1. Relationship between lactate and power.

elicits an average power slightly higher than LT, probably closer to maximal lactate steady state (MLSS), which is the highest power you can maintain without a constant rise in lactate in your blood. However, it is close enough for our purposes here.)

In terms of running, put on the GPS and do the same. In fact, you may not even need to go for a whole hour; a 10K run flat out will get you pretty close to pace at MLSS.[3] For swimming, get in the pool and swim a 3000.[4,5] Then, you can use a little math to calculate the power output for the test. Piece of cake, right?

Yeah, right. Getting athletes to regularly test themselves for an hour is kind of like trying to shove a Twinkie into a parking meter. It just doesn't work.

How to solve this problem? Your next best option is figuring our your Critical Power or Critical Velocity. Please do not confuse the scientific term **C**ritical **P**ower (the important one that you need to know about) with the "critical power" or "cp" popularized by certain coaches (which you don't need to know about unless you want to confuse people). I will explain the difference below.

Critical **P**ower (the real one): A scientific term developed by Dr. Monod in the early 1960's, Critical Power describes the work - time relationship, and permits you to attempt to differentiate between aerobic (the kind of power that would predominate in a long race) and anaerobic work capacity (the kind of power that would predominate in short sprint of a few seconds).[6] Critical Power is a way of comparing your work capacity for different periods of time to discover the power that you could maintain for "a long time". In point of fact, it is a good way of estimating 1 hour power and is close enough for our purposes. (In our experience, it tends to overestimate 1-hour power by just a little bit, especially in amateur athletes.)[7]

> **Power at LT ≈ 1 hour best power ≈ Critical Power ≈ Power at MLSS ≈ FTP ≈ "Threshold Power"**

CHAPTER 2
Watt's Hard? Watt's Easy? Setting the Benchmark

You figure out Critical Power by making a graph of your work capacity at 3 minutes and 20 minutes, and then finding the slope of the line that connects them. In fact, there are software packages that will calculate it for you (I wrote two of them, RaceDay and TriUtilities).

1. One day when feeling spunky, do an short, all-out interval that lasts about 3 minutes.
2. On another day, do a long, all-out interval that lasts about 20 minutes.
3. Type these intervals into the Critical Power calculator in TriUtilities or RaceDay.
4. Voila.

If you don't have RaceDay or TriUtilities, here's how you do it using a calculator. Let's assume you did 320 watts for the 3 minute test, and 240 for the 20 minute test.

1. Multiply your average power for the short interval by the number of seconds in the interval. For instance: 320 watts x 180 seconds = 57,600 joules.
2. Multiply your average power for the long interval by the number of seconds in the interval. For instance: 240 watts x 1200 seconds = 288,000 joules.
3. Divide the difference in the joules by the difference in the seconds. For instance: (288,000-57,600) / (1200-180) = 225.88 watts = Critical Power.

Now for the *other* critical power...

critical power (fake): Used by certain coaches to mean the maximal power you can maintain for different durations of time. For instance, your "CP 30" would be the best power you could maintain for 30 minutes. You should NOT use this term. A better term

> **Critical Power (CP)** - A way of comparing your work capacity for different periods of time to discover the power you could maintain for "a long time". Highly correlated with power at LT.

would be "30 minute maximal power", which is descriptive and does not bastardize accepted scientific terminology. We will never mention the fake critical power again.

Of course, it can be difficult to wrap your head around the idea of Critical Power when talking about running and swimming. Because of this, you can instead calculate Critical Velocity. It works just the same as Critical Power.

Let's assume you did a run test protocol, and covered 1000M in 4 minutes for the short test, and 5000M in 20 minutes for the long test.

1. Subtract the meters for the short test from the number of meters for the long test. For example, 5000-1000 = 4000M.
2. Subtract the number of seconds for the short test from the number of seconds for the long test. For instance, 1200 - 240 = 960.
3. Divide the difference in meters by the difference in seconds. For instance: 4000 / 960 = 4.166 meters / second = Critical Velocity = The speed you could probably hold for about 10K.

You can do the same thing for swimming. Short test, long test, subtract, divide and you now know the speed you can hold for about 3000M.

No matter how you choose to test yourself or your athletes, the most important thing you can do is be consistent. Run the test the exact same way, every time, and on the same course / turbo trainer, or in the same pool if possible, and under the same environmental conditions. We are already trying to make an estimate of this elusive "threshold" power or pace. Don't make matters worse by using different kinds of tests each month, or doing the test differently each month, and introducing the possibility of more error.

You'll want to keep your CP / CV in mind when you are training and racing, especially as the distance you need to go increases. The reason for this is that below CP / CV, your exercise capacity is primarily limited by the fatigue resistance of your muscles. Above CP / CV, your exercise capacity becomes limited by a number of things, including the amount of carbohydrate your body has on board. Thus, if you are performing a workout or race that lasts longer than an hour, but are spending a lot of time at a power output or velocity that is higher than what you know you can do for an hour, you are setting yourself up for fatigue and lackluster performance.

Now, Critical Power / Power at LT or MLSS is one important benchmark to keep in mind. The other really important benchmark to keep in mind is power output or pace at VO2max. Simply put, VO2max is the maximum volume of oxygen that can be used by the body during exhaustive exercise. Since power output and oxygen use rise together, and since we don't have a good way of measuring oxygen use without a laboratory and a lot of expensive machines, we can think in terms of power output at VO2max.

VO2max is primarily determined by the maximal pumping capacity of the heart. The more blood you can move around, the more muscle cells can be used at any one time and the more power you can generate. It in the purest sense, it is probably the best measure of cardiovascular fitness. A very well trained athlete can maintain VO2max for about 5-12 minutes. This would be akin to an athlete running about 3K on the track, or swimming 300-800M in the pool, with the understanding that these efforts would be all-out, eye-ball bulging affairs where you start out afraid that you are going to drop dead, and end up hoping that you actually will die and end the pain.

You can guesstimate power at VO2max (pVO2max) or velocity at VO2max (vVO2max) using a variation of something called the University of Montreal Track Test. I discuss this particular test in

> ## The University of Montreal Track Test
>
> **Figure out your vVO2max for running.**
> 1. Run on a track (or with a GPS receiver) at a speed of 8.5 km/hr.
> 2. Accelerate by 1 km/hr every 2 minutes.
> 3. The fastest speed you can hold for the entire 2 minutes without slowing down is your vVO2max.
>
> **Figure out your pVO2max for cycling.**
> 1. Ride on a quiet road on a day with little wind at an easy pace, or on a trainer with a power meter.
> 2. Raise power output by 20 watts every 2 minutes.
> 3. The highest power you can sustain for the entire 2 minutes without fading is your pVO2max.
>
> **Figure out your vVO2max for swimming.**
> 1. Bring a helper and a stopwatch to the pool.
> 2. Swim at your easiest pace.
> 3. Accelerate by 5-10 seconds/100M every 2 minutes. Have your helper signal you when you need to speed up. Your helper should record your 25 meter splits.
> 4. Your helper should signal you to stop when you are no longer maintaining pace. Your fastest sustained 2 minute speed is your vVO2max.
>
> Adapted from: Leger and Boucher. An indirect running multistage field test, the Universite de Montreal Track Test. *Can J Appl Sports Sci*; 5: 77-84, 1980.

Scientific Training for Triathletes. If you don't have the book, see above for the protocol.

Now, VO2max and Critical Power / Critical Velocity go hand in hand. If VO2max sets the absolute limit of aerobic performance, Critical Power / Critical Velocity is an indicator of how much of that maximum ability you can use in a triathlon or other long endurance task. Think of it like a house. The ceiling is the Critical Power, the top of the attic is VO2max, and the roof is you peak power output. The more space you have between critical power and

CHAPTER 2
Watt's Hard? Watt's Easy? Setting the Benchmark

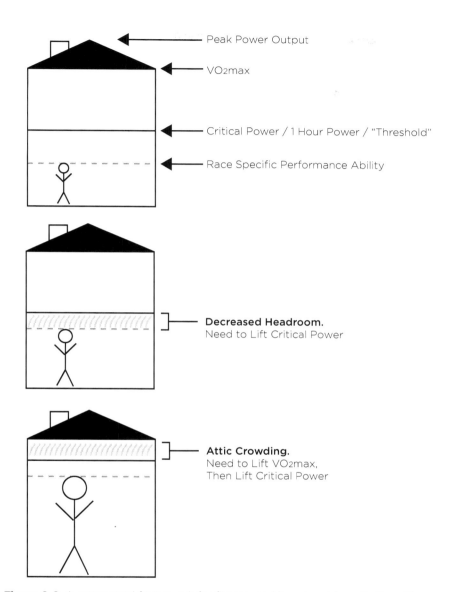

Figure 2-2. A conceptual framework for fitness, and how to address limiters. The athlete's physical condition is equal to the height of the stick figure.

power at VO2max (the ceiling and the attic), the easier your race efforts feel.

To extend this analogy a bit, let's imagine that your fitness or current race power is equal to your height (Figure 2-2). You walk into your house, and mark your height on the wall. With time, as you train, you grow taller. In the beginning, the house grows with you. However, what you will find is that with time you will begin to bump your head on the ceiling. You need to do some specific construction on the house to raise the ceiling so that you can continue to grow. However, what you will quickly find is that you are squeezing the ceiling too close to the attic above. Eventually, you need to raise the attic as well.

You can see what I am driving at here. Your performance has certain limiters (LT and VO2max), and if you want to keep getting better, you need to specifically address these limiters. If you don't, you are setting yourself up to have the same performances year after year. Of course, this begs the question, "How do I specifically target these limiters?" Good question. We will get into that shortly.

CHAPTER 3
Plyometrics: Explosive Exercise To Develop Power

There is a lot of confusion, particularly in the lay press and particularly in endurance sports with regard to the need for strength. If you read *Scientific Training for Triathletes*, you already understand that the scientific literature runs 3:1 to 4:1 against strength training being of any benefit to endurance athletes. The reason for this is rather simple: strength is about generating force, for example, a maximal leg press effort of 500 pounds. However, during endurance exercise, we are operating far below our maximal strength capacity. Thus, the problem isn't strength per se, but *power*. The athlete must be able to do much less than their maximal possible force production, but they must be able to do it rapidly, and for a long period of time. The task feels hard, and our brain *erroneously* assumes the problem is strength, because we have a hard time differentiating between strength and power.

All that said, there are times in swimming, cycling, and running where the ability to generate pure force, that is, the athlete's strength, really is important. For instance, a track cyclist doing a standing start, or a swimmer or track sprinter coming out of the blocks. Even in this case, though, it is critical that the force be applied explosively. Remember the word *explosive*. It is the key to doing the type of strength training that may in fact help your endurance performance. We develop explosive strength through the use of something called plyometrics.

CHAPTER 3
Plyometrics: Explosive Exercise To Develop Power

To effectively address plyometrics, we need to bring up specificity. As we discussed in *Scientific Training for Triathletes*, specificity of training is of paramount importance. It means that to get better at something, we need to do that something exactly. Yet, people often do not realize just how finely we must apply the principle. For instance, we might think that by going to the weight room and practicing a lot of squats, we might be able to improve our leg press or leg extension ability, since those lifts use the same muscles. It turns out that this is not true (Figure 3-1). The nervous system adapts to training so specifically that adaptations that improve one activity do not apply as well to other activities that use the same muscle groups.

So, the first thing we must ensure is that our plyometric exercises are sport specific. You can see some examples in the following illustrations. The very first thing you will want to notice is that none of these moves are standard gym-style free weight or machine lifts. Such training is simply not specific enough and the utility of such exercise has been soundly disproved in the literature, as I wrote earlier. (That said, it might not be inadvisable to do some nonspecific weight training in the off season, simply as preparation for the plyometric exercise to come.)

While there has not been a great deal of research into plyometrics, the research that has been done is encouraging, especially with

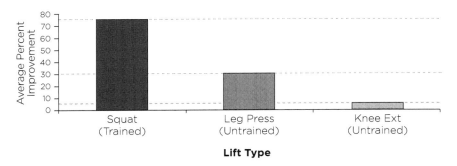

Figure 3-1. Relationship between a trained lift, and untrained lifts that use the same muscles. Note the significant (and perhaps unexpected) differences. Data from Sale (1988), Fahey (1998), and Skiba (unpublished observations).

regard to running.[8,9,10,11] It is thought that plyometrics function by improving the spring-like rebound of the muscles and soft tissues. This likely involves both enhanced stiffness of the tissue itself, and functional stiffness before foot strike as a result of improved reflex arcs that allow better pre-tensioning of the muscle.[12] Case reports in elite athletes, including Paula Radcliffe, the current World Record holder in the women's marathon, indicate a correlation between running economy and stiffness (or rather, loss of flexibility as measured by a sit-and-reach test).[13,14] Theoretically, this permits the athlete to use less oxygen to run at the same speed, because the elastic snap of the muscles and tendons provide some of the energy required.

There is less evidence available with regard to swimming performance, and what evidence there is, is not encouraging. Studies done in sprint (50M) swimmers have repeatedly shown no improvement in 50M time or flip-turn performance.[15,16] There has been some resurgence in interest here, however, as the popular media has reported that Dara Torres relied heavily on plyometric training in the run up to her silver medal performance at the Beijing Olympics in 2008, at the age of 41. Hopefully, this will encourage more research in the area.

Cycling references are also difficult to come by. One reasonable study was done by Bastiaans in 2001, and showed little in the way of performance improvement with explosive weight training. Rather, the results can be best interpreted as saying that it is possible to replace almost 40% of a cyclists training with explosive strength training without a measurable decrease in performance as defined by the study.[17]

It is difficult to develop a best practice as far as this type of training goes, as opinions in the field are largely anecdotal and the proposed mechanisms speculative.[18] For the moment, I believe it is best to limit plyometric training to running exercises. With this in mind, we can attempt to make some calls regarding what sort of plyometric / explosive strength training should work for running.

CHAPTER 3
Plyometrics: Explosive Exercise To Develop Power

These exercises typically involve hopping, skipping or bouncing. I have included a few examples below, and I divide them between "simple plyometric exercises" and "functional plyometric exercises".

These should be performed 3-4 days per week during the appropriate training cycle, for perhaps 20 minutes per session. Norse Olympic Coaches Ronald Klomp and Frans Bosch caution athletes that these exercises are aimed at technique and quickness, not brute force. The movements should be light, as though you are skipping through dry leaves and trying to crush as few as possible. You should be "bouncing".

Plyometric Running Exercises

Progression of Simple Plyometric Exercises

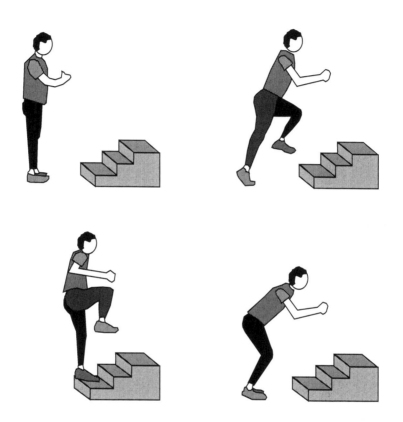

Stair Hopping. From a standing position, and using both feet, jump up and forward onto a step, box or stool, and bounce right back down. Once you have mastered this, make your landing on the box with 1 foot, and jump off with 1 foot, landing on both feet on the ground. Repeat.

CHAPTER 3
Plyometrics: Explosive Exercise To Develop Power

Plyometric Running Exercises *(continued)*

Progression of Simple Plyometric Exercises *(continued)*

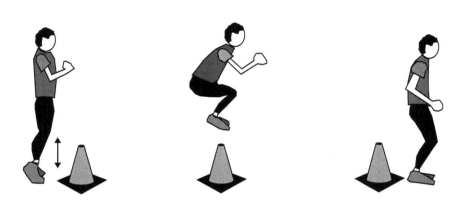

Cone Hopping. From a standing position, bounce once and then spring forward over a cone or other obstacle. Repeat.

CHAPTER 3 | 29
Plyometrics: Explosive Exercise To Develop Power

Progression of Simple Plyometric Exercises *(continued)*

The Box-Jump Cone-Hop. Set up a box or stool with 2 cones in front, spaced a few feet apart. Jump down from the stool, then bounce over the first cone, and then the second cone.

Plyometric Running Exercises *(continued)*

Progression of Functional Plyometric Exercises

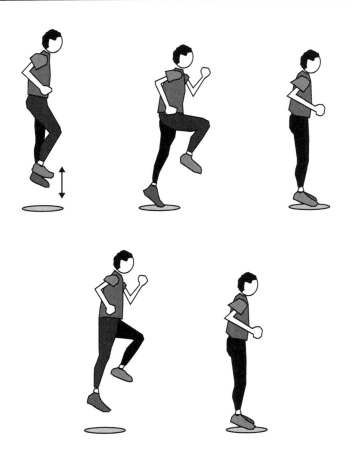

Forward Leap. Once the previous exercises have been mastered, the athlete must advance to training more closely related to functional running mechanics. Bounce once on both feet, then jump forward, taking off from one leg, landing on both feet, then take off with the opposite leg. Once you have mastered this, alternate heights: high, low, high, low.

Progression of Functional Plyometric Exercises (continued)

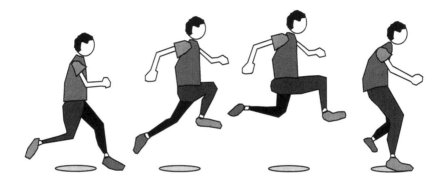

Bounding Repeats. The next step in the functional progression is bounding. Run several steps, and jump off one leg. Run several more steps, then jump off the opposite leg. Repeat.

CHAPTER 3
Plyometrics: Explosive Exercise To Develop Power

Plyometric Running Exercises *(continued)*

Progression of Functional Plyometric Exercises *(continued)*

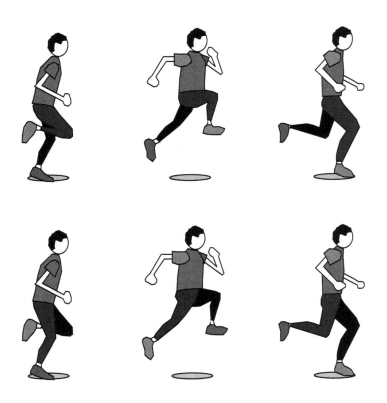

Triple Jump. Run 5-6 steps, then jump off one leg, land on the opposite leg, then take off from this leg, and repeat 3x per leg. Once mastered, this can progress to uphill bounding on a gentle slope, perhaps a 2-3% grade.

---

* Please note that this listing not all inclusive. There are innumerable similar exercises you can design yourself, or find demonstrated elsewhere. An excellent reference is Bosch and Klomp's *Running: Biomechanics and Exercise Physiology Applied in Practice* (Elsevier Churchill Livingstone, 2005). It's worth your while to get a copy, as it is without question the best work in the field.

CHAPTER 4
Zones: The Specifics of Training

By this time, you have almost certainly heard of the concept of "training by zones". Intuitively, it makes sense. If we really believe that the body has a number of different aspects to it's physiology, it stands to reason that there may be more or less efficient ways of training those aspects.

Now, it is important to realize that zones are man made. Your body doesn't know one zone from another. To your physiology, all of the zones sort of "smear" together. In other words, doing long intervals at Critical Power will really help improve your 1-hour best power, but they will also help you at higher power outputs, at least a little. Likewise, doing lots of long distance training will make you more fatigue resistant, but this type of training will also help improve your Critical Power, at least a little bit.

Thus, the reason we set up zones is so that we narrow things down a little. It permits us to be time-efficient, and design workouts that focus *primarily* on one thing or another. However, we need to understand that these workouts don't *actually* focus on just that one thing.

The following chart is taken from *Scientific Training for Triathletes*. In this chart, you will note that I have added Zone VI to the mix. This is largely, but not entirely irrelevant to to the training of most triathletes in most race situations, particularly in the United States. (The most notable exception would be athletes who participate in draft legal / ITU racing, or in races with multiple very short,

Training Zones

Exercise power and/or pace and expected physiologic adaptations.

Zone I	Recovery
%LTHR	<69%
%LT Swim Pace	>107%
%LT Run Pace	>125%
%VO2max Run Pace	>135%
%LT Power	<56%
Key Concept(s)	Promotion of circulation, glycogen restoration and repair; *rest without inactivity.*
Specific Adapt.	None

Zone II	Endurance
%LTHR	69-83%
%LT Swim Pace	107-103%
%LT Run Pace	124-115%
%VO2max Run Pace	134-125%
%LT Power	56-75%
Key Concept(s)	Improvement of slow twitch fiber fatigue resistance; *Length more important than intensity.*
Specific Adapt.	Minimal improvement in oxidative enzyme levels Minimal improvement in LT Minimal Improvement in glycogen storage capacity Minimal conversion of Type IIx to Type IIa fibers

Zone III	Tempo
%LTHR	69-83%
%LT Swim Pace	103-101%
%LT Run Pace	114-105%
%VO2max Run Pace	124-115%
%LT Power	76-90%
Key Concept(s)	Long race pace training: Marathon/IM/Half-IM. *Do not spend significant time here unless racing longer events.*
Specific Adapt.	Maximal improvement in glycogen storage capacity Moderate improvement in oxidative enzyme levels Moderate improvement in LT Moderate conversion of Type IIx to Type IIa fibers Minimal improvement in Type I hypertrophy Minimal improvement in muscle capillarization Minimal improvement in cardiac output Minimal improvement in VO2max Minimal improvement in plasma volume

CHAPTER 4
Zones: The Specifics of Training

Zone IV	LT
%LTHR	95-105%
%LT Swim Pace	101-98%
%LT Run Pace	104-95%
%VO2max Run Pace	114-105%
%LT Power	91-105%
Key Concept(s)	Maximize metabolic fitness of muscles; *critical for all endurance race distances.*
Specific Adapt.	Maximal improvement in LT Maximal improvement in oxidative enzyme levels Moderate improvement in glycogen storage capacity Moderate conversion of Type IIx to Type IIa fibers Moderate improvement in cardiac output Moderate improvement in VO2max Moderate improvement in plasma volume Minimal improvement in Type I hypertrophy Minimal improvement in muscle capillarization

Zone V	VO2max
%LTHR	>106%
%LT Swim Pace	98-92%
%LT Run Pace	94-84%
%VO2max Run Pace	104-95%
%LT Power	106-120% or measured power at VO2max +/- 5%
Key Concept(s)	Maximize cardiac fitness; *important for all endurance race distances.*
Specific Adapt.	Maximal improvement in VO2max Maximal improvement in cardiac output Maximal increased plasma volume Moderate improvement in muscle capillarization Moderate improvement in Type I hypertrophy Minimal conversion of Type IIx to Type IIa fibers Minimal improvement in oxidative enzyme levels Minimal improvement in glycogen storage capacity

Zone VI	Anaerobic Capacity
%LTHR	N/A
%LT Swim Pace	<92%
%LT Run Pace	<84%
%VO2max Run Pace	<95%
%LT Power	>120%
Key Concept(s)	Maximize anaerobic capacity; *important in select race / tactical situations.*
Specific Adapt.	Maximal improvement in anaerobic capacity

Data from: Daniels (1998), Coggan (2003), Billat (2000, 2003).

CHAPTER 4
Zones: The Specifics of Training

very steep climbs.) Be this as it may, the important thing to note is that this Zone VI really isn't based on your Critical Power / Critical Velocity. Why?

It's like this: The shorter and harder your effort, the less it has to do with your aerobic fitness. An all out effort of perhaps 90 seconds is roughly a 50/50 split between aerobic and anaerobic energy sources. It makes little sense to score much shorter efforts in relation to your Critical Power / Critical Velocity. Rather, it makes more sense to view these efforts in terms of your personal best for the duration in question. For example, if (for whatever reason) you needed to have a high 1-minute power output, it would make sense to test your 1-minute best power output and then decide if this was good enough or if it needed addressing.

The next thing you should note is that the percentages of Critical Velocity / "threshold" velocity (i.e. about 3000M velocity) are slightly different for swimming. In other words, the easy zone for swimming is around 94% of Critical Velocity, and the space between zones is much tighter. One of the reasons for this is that water is about 800x more dense than air. Thus, every increase in speed requires a larger increase in power output than you might expect (Figure 4-1).

What you can see here is that traveling at 90-94% of your

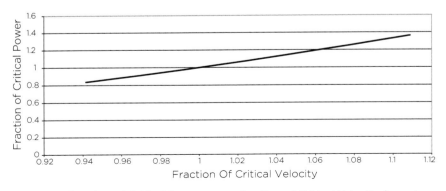

Figure 4-1. Fraction of Critical Power versus fraction of Critical Velocity for swimming. Note that small increases in velocity require large increases in power.

Critical Velocity / 3000M pace (relatively easy swimming) requires you to use only 80% of the power it takes you to reach Critical Velocity. Look what happens when you try to speed up to Critical Velocity, which is less than a 10% increase in speed. The power requirement goes up by almost 20%! As you can see from the shape of the curve, this difference gets larger the faster you ago. Again, this is the reason why we use time and speed for pacing, but we want to think in terms of power because that better reflects the stress we are under during exercise.

Let's talk in a bit more detail about addressing specific systems with specific training, and let's think about training in the simplest way possible. As we discussed previously, we know that to improve at something, we need to work at it exactly. For instance, if we wanted to get better at shooting foul shots in basketball, we'd stand at the foul line and practice for many hours. It might be more fun to work on that skyhook, but we couldn't expect it to help our foul shooting very much. Likewise, it makes sense that if we want to improve our power output at VO2max, we'd spend time doing intervals at that power output. Let's tackle that chart zone by zone, and discuss workout possibilities for one of my typical age group triathletes. Please reference the following charts for pace information.

Swim

Zone	Low End Pace	High End Pace
Zone 1 - Recover	2:00/100M	1:56/100M
Zone 2 - Easy	1:56/100M	1:54/100M
Zone 3 - Tempo	1:54/100M	1:50/100M
Zone 4 - Threshold	1:50/100M	1:48/100M
Zone 5 - VO2	1:48/100M	1:44/100M
Zone 6 - AC	1:44+/100M	N/A

CHAPTER 4
Zones: The Specifics of Training

Bike

Zone	Low End Power	High End Power
Zone 1 - Recover	0W	142W
Zone 2 - Easy	142W	191W
Zone 3 - Tempo	194W	229W
Zone 4 - Threshold	232W	268W
Zone 5 - VO$_2$	270W	306W
Zone 6 - AC	306W+	N/A

Run

Zone	Low End Pace	High End Pace
Zone 1 - Recover	0	9:00/mile (5:36/K)
Zone 2 - Easy	9:00/mile (5:36/K)	8:00/mile (4:58/K)
Zone 3 - Tempo	8:00/mile (4:58/K)	7:30/mile (4:40/K)
Zone 4 - Threshold	7:30/mile (4:40/K)	7:00/mile (4:21/K)
Zone 5 - VO$_2$	7:00/mile (4:21/K)	6:45/mile (4:12/K)
Zone 6 - AC	6:45/mile (4:12/K)+	N/A

Examples and Explanations
Of Targeted Training

Zone I: Recovery

Recovery isn't training. It's recovery. The fact of the matter is that many of us train because we like doing it (or because we are obsessed). Thus, what we want to do is be able to recover without resorting to absolute inactivity. We don't expect training in this zone to do anything for us. It is simply something to do with our legs while on the way to a coffee shop or something.

Example Workouts:
Swim: 1500M easy, done as a descending ladder 500-400-300-200-100 at ≈ 2:00 / 100M on 1:00 rest
Bike: 1 hour @ 135 watts. Avoid hills.
Run: 40 minutes @ about 5:30 / K.

Zone II: Endurance

Long endurance training is an important part of any program. Here, the primary adaptation we are looking for is improving the fatigue resistance of the slow-twitch muscle fibers. This sort of training should often include periods of directed tempo riding to induce more metabolic adaptations, or just reduce boredom. For long course athletes, these sessions should always include long periods (10-30 minutes at a time) of tempo effort training, since they will be racing in that tempo range.

It is important to remember that this type of training isn't easy per se. It is directed, long training. It should require a little bit of concentration to maintain this power or pace.

Example Workouts:
Swim: 3000M Total
Main set = 3 x 500 @ 1:54 / 100M on 0:20 rest interval
Bike: 4 hours @ 160 to 170W. Include 3 x 10 minutes of tempo riding at 200-210W. Keep hills any hills under 95% of Critical Power.
Run: Run 10K @ 5:30 / K. Maintain a constant level of exertion going over hills, which may require you to slow down slightly.

Zone III: Tempo

Tempo riding is the meat and potatoes of most long course triathlon training. The reason for this is that it is close enough to the Threshold zone to help raise LT / Critical Power, however, it lacks the higher recovery cost of Threshold / Zone IV training. This is often referred to as "Sweet Spot Training". For sprint and Olympic distance training, tempo training should be minimized in favor of Zone IV / Threshold training as it is more specific to the demands of the race.

Example Workouts:

Swim: 2500M Total
Main set = 3 x 400M @ 1:54 / 100M on 1:00 recovery interval
Bike: 3 hours at 160-170W. Include 3 x 30 minutes of tempo riding at 200-210W.
Run: 1 hour total, include 4 x 1 mile at 4:48 / K

Zone IV: Threshold

These workouts are typically quite difficult. The goal is to maximize the metabolic fitness of the muscles, and raise sustainable power output. I usually don't write the total session longer than 1 to 1.5 hours for age groupers, and I never write the work interval for longer than about 20 minutes. In age groupers, it is often advisable to begin by building these workouts in multiples of 5 minutes on 1-2 minute rest, i.e. 4 x 5 minutes at CP with 2 minutes of recovery between, then decrease the rest interval over a period of a few weeks until they are able to hold 20 minutes straight, and then continue by adding another 4 x 5 minute segment and again decreasing the rest until they are able to do 2 x 20 minutes on 2-5 minutes recovery.

Please take special note of the fact that these are not 20 minute intervals at the best power you can hold for 20 minutes. These are 20 minute intervals at the best pace you could hold for about an hour. The work should be difficult, but by no means excruciating. If it is, or if the athlete cannot hold power for the duration, that is a good sign that you've set the zone too high and you need to back off.

Example Workouts:

Swim: 3000M Total
Main set: 4 x 300M @ 1:48 / 100M on 1:00 rest interval
Bike: 1 hour at 170W, with 2 x 20 minutes at 250W on 2:00 rest.
Run: 45 minutes total, main set = 3 x 1 mile at 4:30 / K

Another important point to consider is the training status and ability of the athlete. A nice review of the literature was undertaken by Londeree in 1997.[19] Based on his analysis, he concluded that training at or near lactate threshold was sufficient stimulus to improve LT, however, better athletes require a more severe stimulus to realize gains. This makes intuitive sense as well, and it has certainly been borne out in the way I've trained professional athletes. A reasonable way of addressing the issue in better trained athletes is the over-under interval. You can adapt the interval for different sports quite easily. The way to do it is to begin the work interval in high Zone IV, build to a power output or pace in the lowest region of Zone V over the course of a couple of minutes, and then maintain it for 5 minutes or more. As fatigue begins to set in, drop down into Zone IV. Then, repeat it.

Recall the house analogy we discussed earlier. You need to look at your threshold power / pace, which is the ceiling, and your VO2max power / pace, which is the attic. In elite athletes, I've sometimes found the two are close enough together that it is difficult to raise the ceiling without crowding the attic above. In this case, it may be advisable to place a greater emphasis on VO2max training for a short time in an effort to expand the space between before again addressing threshold power.

This is one of those situations where a combination of art and science is appropriate. I can't give you an exact recipe. If you are pushing threshold level work without success, and find that the over/under approach is coming up dry as well, it may be time to change it up. It is certainly worthwhile trying as it has been demonstrated that irrespective of initial training status, increasing velocity / power at LT is a major factor in improving time to exhaustion.[20]

Zone V: VO2max

These workouts are typically short and sweet. The idea is to drive the heart rate up near maximum, which forces it to adapt by becoming larger and stronger. They are typically done in a "lather-rinse-repeat" methodology, i.e multiples of a particular interval with equal rest. These sorts of intervals should also help increase the capillary bed in the muscles, allowing better delivery of oxygen to more motor units, although this is likely more important in very highly trained athletes.

In recent years, there has been some interest in what has been come to be known as the "30/30" workout. This idea was most recently studied by Dr. Veronique Billat, although it was apparently first looked at by

Gorostiaga in 1991.[21] The main set of the workout involves running 30 seconds at vVO2max, followed by 30 seconds of easy recovery, repeated many times over. Dr. Billat studied this workout in 2000, comparing to a steady, hard run, and her findings were interesting.[22] Essentially, she showed that the 30/30 allowed runners to maintain a longer period of time at VO2max (8 minutes versus 3 minutes) and to run faster during the workout (by about 1.6 kph). It remains to be seen whether this is actually a superior methodology.

Dr. Billat has also turned up some other interesting results with regard to individualizing the interval program.[23] For instance, it is possible to discover how long you can maintain vVO2max (called TlimvVo2max) by running on a treadmill at that speed until you can no longer continue. This known, you then design your interval workout by writing the interval length as 50% of your TlimvVo2max, and do 5 repetitions with equal rest. The training program also included a 2 x 20 minute threshold session weekly. This improved vVO2max significantly. The interesting thing was that increasing the number of these interval sessions to 3 per week did not further improve performance. Thus, one such session is likely sufficient.

Although VO2 workouts can seem very difficult in the moment, athletes usually recover from them fairly quickly, provided that they run at the prescribed pace, and not "all out", and that they are careful to finish feeling as though they still had one or two repetitions in them. The point of these sessions is to deliver a directed stimulus to force the adaptation you are interested in, not crawling off the track so that you can brag about the killer set you just finished as your kid tows you home in their little radio flyer wagon.

Example Workouts:
Swim: 2000M Total
Main set: 10 x 100M @ 1:44 / 100M on 1:00 rest interval
Bike: 1 hour at 170W, with 5 x 3 minutes at 290-300W on 3 minutes rest.
Run: 45 minutes total, main set = 4 x 800M at 4:10 / K pace

Zone VI: Anaerobic Capacity

Much of the energy supplied by the muscles in this zone is derived from "nonrenewable" (at least, nonrenewable in the short term) sources. Allow me to explain briefly. The universal energy currency of the body is called adenosine triphosphate (ATP). You can make it from both sugar and fat. When you need energy to do something, the muscle cell splits off one of the phosphates, which leaves you with adenosine diphosphate (ADP). The body then slaps another phosphate back onto the ADP to make ATP, provided it has the means to do so, so that it can be recycled and provide more energy for muscle contraction.

During sudden, high intensity exercise, the body doesn't have time to really ramp up metabolism to meet the demand for ATP. Thus, as the muscle cells break down the ATP you have on hand into ADP, they must resort to using local stores of high energy phosphate (i.e. creatine phosphate) to regenerate the ATP. Eventually, you tap out the high energy phosphate stores, feel severe fatigue, and pack it in.

Going to this well is often referred to as "burning a match". It can happen during the mass start of a triathlon swim as you try to jockey into a good position, cover an attack during a draft legal bike leg, or have to out-sprint someone to the finish line. The point is, these sorts of things don't happen very often given the racing that most triathletes do, especially in the United States. Thus, I wouldn't be too worried about doing much of this type of training unless you are really on the pointy end of the field.

If you do feel the need to do this sort of work, it helps to do it with a specific goal in mind. For instance, let's say you need to make the front pack on the swim. The appropriate way to attack the problem would be to go to a couple of similar races and observe your competition. How long do they throw the smack down before settling into their actual race pace, and how fast are they going while they do it? Once you have this information, you can set up a workout to address exactly the kind of power / pace you need to address.

If you are racing a triathlon with a draft legal bike leg (for example, an ITU race or the Desoto Triple T), it may be important to you to be able to stay with a pack over a given hill. Again, do your homework and find out how many watts it will take you to maintain race speed over a hill of that grade. (There are websites that can help you do this.) Structure a workout where you maintain this specific power for the necessary duration.

There are other reasons to do this kind of training. For example, noted exercise physiologist and coach Dr. Jack Daniels regularly prescribes these sorts of intervals during track workouts to improve speed and economy, and while it might be of more benefit to a 1500M or 3K runner, it probably doesn't hurt to do a little bit. It is important to take plenty of recovery between. You should bag the session if they begin to feel really stressful, or if you fall off the pace by more than a few percent.

Example Workouts:

Swim: 2000M Total
Main set: 10 x 100M @ 1:39 / 100M pace on 1:00 rest interval.

Bike: 1 hour at 170W, with 4 x 1 minute at 425W on 5 minutes rest.

Run: 45 minutes total, main set = 8 x 200M at 47s with 400M easy recovery jog between.

You have probably noticed by now that while I have descriptive terms for zones, each workout always comes with a power or pace target that is quite specific. The reason for this is that zones are descriptive more than prescriptive. In other words, while anything more than about 5% over LT power / pace might be slightly better classified as a VO2max workout, the zone is much too broad to be useful. We shouldn't noodle about in a zone aimlessly. This approach still returns results in amateurs who are relatively new to the sport, but if you have been at it for any length of time, you need to have an exact goal in mind. Thus, when we say we are going to run VO2max pace intervals, we run them at about 3K pace, or at the pace we discovered by testing for VO2max pace (i.e. the University of Montreal Track Test). When we say we are riding tempo intervals on the bike and we are planning on racing an iron distance race, we shoot for goal race power.

The important thing to remember is that you want to have very specific ideas about what you are trying to address when you write your workouts. You are going to get the best results when you accurately evaluate the demands of a particular race situation and then target those demands in your training.

CHAPTER 5
Understanding Variability and Intensity

Ok, so now we have an idea of what is hard (going out to train, killing yourself for an hour, and then calling your mom crying), and why it is hard (it's pretty close to your LT), and why that is important to know (LT is the best predictor of how good you are as a triathlete). We know how to write some pretty challenging workouts as well. The next question you ought to be asking yourself is, "How do we compare different kinds of hard?" Riding 2 hours at tempo power is challenging, but so is riding 55 minutes at threshold power. What we would like to be able to do is compare across different types of workouts and find the common thread: what effect did it have on your physiology?

Let's start with a pretty simple case that anyone can relate to. For instance, let's say I asked you to ride an hour as hard as possible on a flat course, and you recorded an average power of 300 watts. Now, if I told you to do the same thing on a hilly course, you'd get a much lower number, perhaps more like 225 watts.

We have a problem here. Both efforts made you want to call your mom and cry. However, your power meter is telling you the second one was WAY easier, and you know this is not true! What you have noticed here are 2 separate, but related problems: *variability* and *intensity*.

First, let's talk about variability. You rode up those hills, and then you coasted the downhills. So, we explained the low watts right there...a lot of zeros got averaged into your file. However, while you

CHAPTER 5
Understanding Variability and Intensity

are coasting, you are still "feeling" what you did on that uphill (i.e. the burn in your thighs). For your body, then, this isn't an on-again, off-again deal. When you started climbing, it wasn't so bad, but a minute or two in, it started to suck. When you hit the downhill, your legs continued to tell you they were unhappy for a while. (A long while, if you are anything like me!) You can see how this works in Figure 5-1.

Now, let's talk about intensity. When riding up those hills, you were burying yourself. You went harder on the uphill than you did on the flats. Those hard efforts are way above your threshold power. As efforts get harder, their impact gets exponentially greater. Think of this in terms of that lactate curve from earlier. As you step up to higher and higher power outputs, each little step is significantly harder than the previous step.

What we would like to do is have a way of weighting your power output, so that we took into account variability (periods of hard effort vs. periods of coasting) and intensity (making the hard efforts exponentially harder, the way your body feels them). I have done this for you by developing the **xPower (XP)** system, although there are other systems on the market. The concept itself was first developed by Dr. Andrew Coggan, the trademark rights to which he later sold (the actual calculation is public domain). The mathematics were validated in two separate studies, one of which was done by yours truly.[24] xPower differs somewhat in how the power data is smoothed. My research shows that both systems work well, and I primarily rely on my system to avoid conflicts with other industry players who have licensed his work. (I have kept XP entirely open source for non-commercial use. You can write your own program to calculate it if you have some free time on your hands.)

The mathematics are usually not particularly important to Joe Triathlete, but it is basically a three step process, and we include it here to make sure the concept is clear to those who are interested.

CHAPTER 5 | 47
Understanding Variability and Intensity

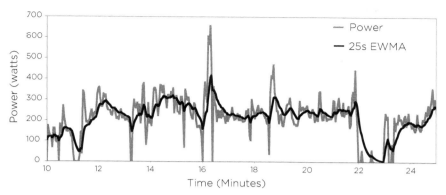

Figure 5-1. Power output and 25 second EWMA of power output.

Step 1: Smooth the power data using an exponentially weighted moving average. This makes sense because your body does lots of things on an exponential basis. This takes care of the on-again, off-again problem we talked about above (Figure 5-1).

Note the difference between what this athlete did (light) and the time course of the physiologic response to the effort (dark). You could think of the dark line as an indicator of how the workout "looks" to the body. It takes a little while to notice a big spike in power output. Look at the difference between the tallest light point and the tallest dark point. Now, look at where the light curve drops to zero, but the dark curve more falls more slowly. See what we are driving at here? You do something, but it takes your physiology a while to figure out what is going on and either ramp itself up significantly or chill out a little.

Step 2: Raise the smoothed power values to the 4th power, to account for the fact that the hard efforts have much more physiologic impact than the easy efforts (Figure 5-2).

Note the difference between the smoothed power (light line, but here it is shown as a fraction of Critical Power, where 1 = 100% of CP) and how that power is weighted in terms of it's physiologic impact on your body (dark line). If we say the light line is how the

CHAPTER 5
Understanding Variability and Intensity

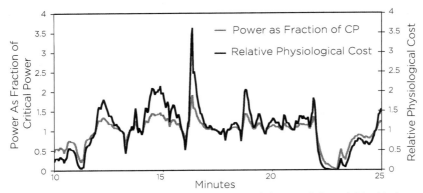

Figure 5-2. 25 second EWMA of power (light) and the way it is weighted in terms of how it "feels" to the body (dark).

workout *looks* to your body, the dark line is how it *feels* to your body. At moderate power outputs, there isn't a huge difference. However, as power climbs, you can see that the impact increases dramatically. This is because the impact of a workout rises with the 4th power of intensity. Again, if you do your 30-minute workout but double how intense the workout is, you have increased it's impact *by many times*. What you are looking at is the reason hard training seems to have a more dramatic impact on fitness, and why you can do less (time-wise), more intense training in order to gain some of the benefits of a greater amount of easy training.

Step 3: Average the weighted power values in Step 2, and take the 4th root. This leaves you with a power value that is both *corrected for variability and corrected for intensity* (Figure 5-3).

The question is, how does this shake out in the end? What have we gained? As it turns out, something very useful. Take a look at Figure 5-3. Both files analyzed are from the same rider. The top panel is from an all-out, 1-hour time trial on a flat course. The second is from an all-out TT on a hilly course.

Look at the horizontal lines. The solid line is the xPower for the effort. The dashed line is the average power. For the flat time trial (top panel), you see that AP and XP end up very close. The effort was not very variable, so either metric is a good description of the effort. In the hilly time trial (bottom panel) you can see the effort is highly variable, and the AP (dashed) seems very low. However, the XP is higher. If you look at the XP between the two graphs, you see that it is about the same. In other words, the xPower allows you to look at two very different rides and ask the question, "Did these two rides "cost" the same, physiologically speaking?"

As you may have guessed, we can apply these same principles to running and swimming, because we can calculate power output for those sports using computer software (e.g. RaceDay). In this case, we can look at power and xPower, but we can also look at pace and

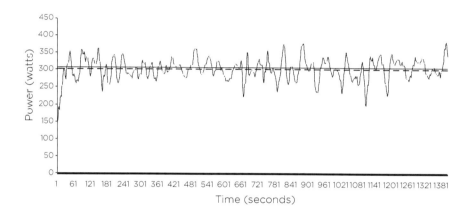

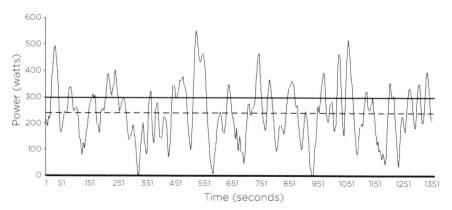

Figure 5-3. Average power (dashed line) and xPower (solid line) for a flat time trial and a hilly time trial undertaken at maximal effort, respectively.

xPace, which is simply the pace after correction for variability and intensity.

What it boils down to is this: If you are riding a **flat ride** or doing a flat run with a relatively **constant power** output, **average power and average pace** are a good descriptors of the requirements. If you are putting out a **highly variable** effort (a very hilly run or training ride, or a criterium), **xPower or xPace** is going to be a better descriptor of the exercise in question.

A nice way of thinking of any given exercise task is in terms of the ratio of xPower to Critical Power. In other words, by dividing the two, we can essentially see what percentage of "threshold effort" any given ride, run, or swim takes. We call this the **Relative Intensity (RI)**. Table 5-1 allows you to ballpark different types of training and the RI you can expect for each.

A RI higher than 1 indicates a supra-threshold effort. If you saw this for a ride longer than 1 hour, it means it is probably time to retest your Critical Power because you are more fit.

The question, of course, is "How necessary is all of this?" Here's the thing: if you look back at some of the research that has been published over the years, you can see that variability in intensity can have a real impact on your ability to perform exercise, even if you don't change how much work you do. For instance, Dr. Noakes and his colleagues did an interesting experiment in the 1990's.[25] They took athletes and made some of them ride at a steady power for a few hours, and then made them do a 20K time trial. They then

Type of workout	Common RI's
Recovery	less than 0.73
Easy	0.73 to 0.83
Tempo	0.83 to 0.93
Threshold	0.93 to 1.03 (for the work interval)
VO2max	1.10+ (for the work interval)
Anaerobic Capacity	Not applicable

Table 5-1. Workout type and corresponding estimated Relative Intensity (RI).

> **Relative Intensity (RI):** Ratio of xPower to Critical power. Indicates the fraction of "threshold effort" the athlete maintained.

added up the number of joules the athletes did (i.e. how much work they did during the steady power segment). In another experiment, they made the athletes do a very variable ride that was just as long as the steady ride. Sometimes they rode hard, and sometimes they rode easy. They made sure the athletes did the same amount of work (i.e. the same number of joules) as the steady ride. Then, they did another 20K time trial.

Here is the interesting thing: the athletes did better in the time trial if it was preceded by steady exercise. If the first exercise task was very variable, with periods of hard work and periods of easy work, the athletes did worse. Why should this be? They did the same amount of work, right?

Remember what we said earlier: the strain of an exercise task, that is, how taxing it is on your body, has much to do with the work *rate*, or *power output*. Thus, when the athletes rode a very variable ride, the periods of the high power output caused more strain on the body, digging into their reserves and leaving them with less in the tank for the subsequent time trial. If you did the appropriate calculations, you'd find that the variable ride had a higher xPower than the steady ride, even though both sets of athletes did the same number of joules of work.

Does the experiment sound familiar at all? You know, doing a lot of riding and then trying to do something hard and / or fast afterwards, like maybe run? *You know, sort of like a triathlon!* Now you are getting the idea. The take home messages are as follows:

⇨ Bike racing is all about getting to the finish line as quickly as possible. The optimal strategy may be to kill yourself on the climbs, because you can puke your guts out on the downhill and collapse at the finish line.

⇨ **Triathlon racing is all about riding fast enough that you don't lose too much time, but slow enough that you can run hard afterwards. As we now see, it is also very much about having an evenly paced effort. Thus, the optimal strategy is most likely not to kill yourself on the climbs, particularly for Olympic through Ultra distance racing.**

We can apply these same principles to running. If you watch a competitive marathon (or triathlon for that matter), you will often see that the front of the pack athletes often throw in surges in pace in an effort to "crack" their competition. What they are doing (possibly without understanding it in the scientific sense) is exploiting the phenomena we saw in Figure 5-3. They do something that incurs a high physiologic cost, raising the xPower for the effort well above the threshold of their competitors in the hopes that they will fatigue more quickly and permit an escape.

CHAPTER 6
How Much Are You Training?
No, *really*.

Ok, so far we have discussed measuring the power for a workout (in watts), how to correct that power if the ride was really hilly / variable (use xPower), and how to decide if a particular workout is hard or easy (look at the Relative Intensity). What we want to do is use this information to figure out a points system for a workout. Then, we could look at different workouts and see how taxing they were on our bodies. As we discussed earlier, this is a better idea than looking at just mileage because it is actually telling us about both how long and how hard the effort was. We do this using something called BikeScore for the bike, SwimScore for swimming and GOVSS (if you have a GPS) / RunScore (if you don't) for running.

You may ask, "Why this is important? Why do I care about measuring the actual amount of training?" That is easy: it turns out that there is a dose / response relationship between exercise and the effect on the athlete. In fact, it is very similar to what you see / expect if you look at a dose of a medication and the body's response to that dose. If you take a little aspirin, your blood gets a little bit thinner. If you take more aspirin, your blood gets even thinner and you may also fix that hangover from your brother's bachelor party. If you take too much aspirin, you'll irritate the lining of your stomach, give yourself a bleeding ulcer and be really, really sick. You can think of the numerical score as the "dose" of exercise instead of medication, or the number of "points" a workout earned you towards your fitness. (We'll talk more about this later).

This concept is not new. In the 1970's, Dr. Eric Banister developed a unit called Training Impulse Score (TRIMPS).[26] It is calculated from a simple equation.

TRIMPS = Exercise duration (minutes) x Average HR (BPM) x An intensity-based weighting factor that is based on HR

If you think about it, this formula makes good sense. We have how long you trained (minutes), we have how hard you trained (how high the HR is), and we also have this weighting factor, which you might have been otherwise puzzled by, but should now understand. This is essentially the same idea we talked about with the lactate curve, which we used to help us understand how much strain increasing power output placed on your body. In fact, Dr. Banister figured out his weighting system by plotting blood lactate against heart rate. The weighting factor is a multiplier that says, in essence "The harder I go, the more difficult it is to go any harder."

Now, we have a problem. If you look at Figure 6-1, you see it goes up to 100%. This makes sense, because your HR can't go any higher than it's maximum. Our issue here is that your heart doesn't

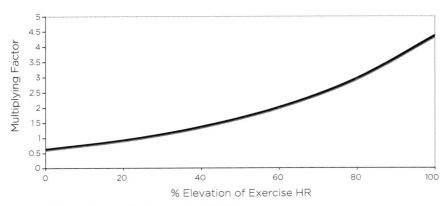

Figure 6-1. Multiplying factor used in TRIMPS.

> **TRIMPS** - The Training Impulse Score is an arbitrary unit that indicates the stress of a workout using heart rate and time.

set the absolute limit. For instance, you may run the 1500M at your maximum heart rate. But, you can also sprint the last 200M. So, now you are traveling faster, which is much more stressful, but you would not know it from looking at your heart rate. It is already redlined. Make sense? So, when you look at the file from your heart rate monitor and calculate your points up, you won't get any "extra credit" for that sprint, even though you buried yourself to do it.

The other problem is this: TRIMPS is based on HR, but your ability to perform, as we discussed earlier, is primarily determined by your lactate threshold. There isn't any really good way to tie HR to LT, because as we also discussed earlier HR can be different day to day even if you are doing exactly the same workout because of temperature changes, sleep patterns, etc.

If we are really interested in knowing exactly what is going on with our training, we want credit for every little bit of every workout. And, we'd also like our points system to be closely tied to the thing that determines our ability to perform, that is, lactate threshold, which we can easily estimate using Critical Power. Fortunately, we can solve both these problems by using power meters for our bikes, pace data for swimming, and GPS or pace for running.

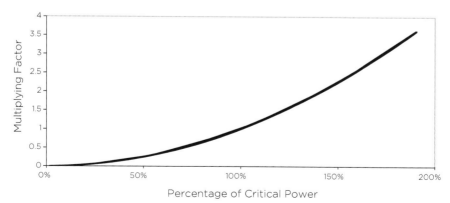

Figure 6-2. Multiplying factor used in the xPower algorithm.

CHAPTER 6
How Much Are You Training? No, *really*.

To start out with, we need a weighting system that makes sense. It would be just like Figure 6-1, except that it also gives you credit for everything you do, even periods of time spent at a power output or speed that is higher than that which would redline your heart rate. It turns out that this is easy. You do just what Dr. Banister did, except instead of making a plot of blood lactate against heart rate, you make it blood lactate against power. Then, we use this to make a multiplying scale where 100% is equal to CP (Figure 6-2).

The next question is, "How do we make a new points scale?"

This part of the story begins with Dr. Andrew Coggan. An avid cyclist and renowned scientist, Dr. Coggan realized the limitations of TRIMPS early on and developed the points system for power meters.[27,28] He used a weighting system just like those we discussed previously. Then, he did something interesting and quite different. He set it up so that the points would be indicative of the effort: 100 points equals 1 hour at threshold power. Thus, this system allows you to compare different workouts nicely. You can, for instance say "My tempo ride of 1 hour and 30 minutes got me 100 points, which is about equal to the number of points I would get from a 70-minute workout with several long intervals at race power." In other words, it gives you a sort of global yardstick you can use to evaluate lots of different rides and understand what their impact was with an easy to digest number.

I did the work to develop analogous systems for running (GOVSS and RunScore) and swimming data (SwimScore), as well as the alternative bike system, BikeScore.[29,30,31,32,33] These systems set 1 hour at Critical Power / Critical Velocity / 1 Hour Power or pace = 100 points.

At the end of the day, the actual score you use is probably irrelevant so long as it takes into account both the duration and intensity of the training, with an important caveat. If you use something like TRIMPS, you need to realize that the score does not adjust itself to your increasing fitness. In other words, if you do a half-hour run today, you may collect 100 TRIMPS. If you do the same run next month, you will again collect 100 TRIMPS. The problem, though, is that you are (or at least, you should be) fitter. Thus, those 100 points don't carry the same weight as the 100 points last month. They don't make you as tired, and they don't add as much to your fitness. You could say that they don't have the same impact.

If you use a metric like BikeScore, which is constantly adjusted based on your fitness, you have a better idea of the impact of your training. For example, let's say you test your Critical Power monthly. This month, it is 200 watts. You do an hour ride at 200 watts, and collect 100 points. Next month, you are fitter, and you find that your critical power has increased to 220 watts. The same 1 hour ride at 200 watts now rightly gains you fewer points...you are fitter, so you should have to train harder to get the same number of points. Make sense?

Now, to address a common misconception: it isn't all about getting the highest score you can. For instance, you can collect 100 points by riding your butt off for an hour, or by riding around easy for a few hours chasing your kids on tricycles. The fact that both tasks gave you the same score is irrelevant. They were so different that we cannot expect they would impact your physiology in the same way. Thus, it isn't all about the points, but the *composition of the points*. A score is meaningful only if you are careful to train in a way that will affect the physiologic systems necessary for you to race well. Therefore, more is not always more, even though some people would like you to think that way.

The last point to keep in mind regarding these scoring systems is that they were devised to relate training to *metabolic* stress. They do not, nor can they, have a lot to do with *mechanical* stress. For instance, running an hour all-out, riding an hour all-out, and swimming an hour all-out have a similar impact on the athlete's working muscles from a metabolic standpoint, but a very different impact from a mechanical standpoint. Running involves eccentric contraction (lengthening against tension) of particular muscles in the legs, which is much more damaging than the concentric contraction (shortening against tension) that primarily makes up swimming and cycling. You can try cooking up various ways of weighting training differently for differently sports (I've tried), but the more you do that, the less the points system it has to do with the metabolic adaptations of training.

In my opinion, you are better off just considering the sports individually, and realizing that there are somewhat different recovery costs for the different sports, and schedule your different workouts differently.

CHAPTER 7

The Nuts and Bolts: Rationally Analyzing Your Training

You now have the background you need in order to intelligently discuss training with power. You understand the difference between the amount of work you do (joules), and how fast you that work (watts). You know certain strength exercises that can help you deliver watts to the road more efficiently (plyometrics and explosive strength training). You know that you should gauge your endurance workouts in reference to our Critical Power or Critical Velocity, because it is very close to power / velocity at LT / MLSS and will be highly correlated with your abilities in short or long races. You know you need to correct your power output if the task you accomplished was very variable (using xPower). Finally you understand that it isn't about distance or time or speed, but scoring workouts in a way that takes into account both the duration and intensity of exercise (using BikeScore, SwimScore, RunScore or GOVSS).

We now need to talk about what to do with your data. Once you have a few rides under your belt, including a race or two and some hard interval workouts of varying duration, it's time to start analyzing your data. The way I would like to approach this in terms of inputs and outputs. Your body is a system that accepts input (training) and produces output (power). Much like a doctor watching what goes into and comes out of a patient, your task is to monitor what is going into the body, and coming out of the body as a result of what went in.

CHAPTER 7
The Nuts and Bolts: Rationally Analyzing Your Training

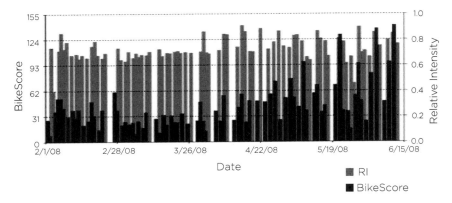

Figure 7-1. Training stress and intensity over the course of a season.

Step 1: Look at the training input in a broad sense

The first thing you need to do is review the composition of training in broad strokes. Here, we are looking at the forest, not necessarily the individual trees. In other words, you want to know how much you are doing, and how hard you are doing it. We'll do this using my software, RaceDay, since it is what I am most familiar with.

Let's start out by looking at the training load and intensity. To begin with, we'll take a look at a good age group athlete, who is doing a pretty standard training build over a period of a few months (Figure 7-1).

You are able to note two things here. First of all, the training load is building. You can see that the athlete's BikeScore (black bars) is trending upwards from February through June. You can also see that the Relative Intensity (gray), that is, what percentage of threshold effort the athlete is maintaining during these workouts, is also increasing. This demonstrates some of the most important principles of training.

1. **Overload:** To improve, you must do more than you did before to force your body to improve.
2. **Adaptation:** The more you do, the more you are able to do.

CHAPTER 7
The Nuts and Bolts: Rationally Analyzing Your Training

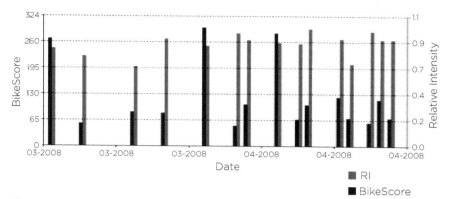

Figure 7-2. Training stress and intensity during a short time window.

Note that the athlete is able to do more and more stressful workouts (higher and higher BikeScores for the biggest days) at higher and higher percentages of threshold effort.

Now, let's zoom in to a much tighter interval. In this case, we will look at a month in the life of an age group iron-distance athlete (Figure 7-2).

The first thing we should notice here is that we have an athlete who is training pretty hard. He is doing a long ride every week that results in a BikeScore of about 260-280, or in the ballpark of an iron-distance bike leg. The Relative Intensity of these sessions is roughly 0.8 to 0.85, well within the tempo range. Now, this is more the sort of RI you would expect for a half-iron race, and there is an important reason for this: you want to have plenty of "overhead" for your race. In other words, if you can put up a BikeScore of 260 at an RI of 0.85, doing the same thing during a race at a more iron-appropriate RI of 0.75 will be no big deal.

Now, look at his shorter rides. These yield a BikeScore of around 60 to 100, or roughly 60 to 100% of the strain incurred by riding an hour at Critical Power. The intensity of those sessions may fall around 0.9 or better, or about 90% of the intensity of an effort of 1 hour at Critical Power.

This is the sort of pattern we often see in a good iron-distance

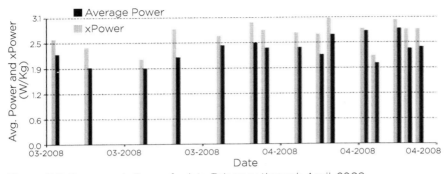

Figure 7-3. Power and xPower for late February through April, 2008.

age group athlete with limited time (in this case, a professional with a busy schedule and a family). There may only be time for 3 workouts a week, but some short / hard stuff combined with a long ride at a reasonable intensity may be good enough to do the job. When time is a limiter, the athlete cannot afford much in the way of long distance training, and must get the maximum bang from their training time by training hard. The take home message is that if you need to go short, you also need to go hard.

Let's stick with this athlete for a moment, so that we can look at what kind of numbers he is putting up in the absolute sense, and how variable the training is, by looking at the average power and xPower (Figure 7-3).

In the purest sense, we are looking at both training and performance here. What we see is that as the month progresses, the athlete is able to push himself from 2.22 W/Kg (first set of bars from left) to a little better than 2.4 W/Kg (5th set of bars from the left on the long ride). We also know this is not a fluke, because he was able to put up similar numbers on April 6th (8th set of bars from the left). We know that on the ride on March 30th (5th set of bars from the left), the xPower and average power are quite close. This indicates that not only has the athlete's ability to produce power improved, he has the ability to do it steadily, which as we discussed earlier is critical for success in triathlon.

Thus, given he is able to generate a BikeScore in the ballpark of what we would see for an iron-distance bike leg at an RI greater than that required for successful iron distance racing, I would expect him to have a reasonable long course performance, provided that he has been doing enough running

Step 2: Look at the performance output in a broad sense

The previous sorts of analysis tell us much about what the athlete has done, and thus the minimum he is capable of doing. Our next question is this: Is the training program effective? Essentially, we ask the computer looks at each file and ask the question, "What is the best power output you ever held for 5 minutes? What about 6 minutes? How about 10 minutes?" You get the idea. You generate a curve that is high on the left (short time periods) and low on the right (long time periods). By looking at your relative performances, you can see where your strengths and weaknesses lie, and look for improvements over time.

Let's start out by looking at a rather general case (Figure 7-4). This data came from an athlete who was coming back from an injury and subsequent surgery. The athlete's coach decided that the program should focus on general fitness improvement, without much in the way of intensity. The idea was to bring the athlete back

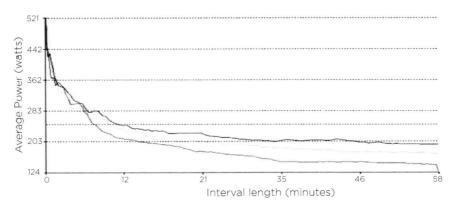

Figure 7-4. Maximum power for an athlete from January-March (gray), April (light gray) and May-June (black). Note the gradual improvement with time.

to the point where he could train properly again.

The gray line is indicative of the best performance an athlete ever had from January through March, the light gray line indicates April, and the dark line indicates May and June.

Looking at this graph, we can see some interesting things. For instance, we can see that the curves almost intersect at the 5-minute mark. Across the beginning of the program, the athlete only improved about 10 watts there. Thus, if the goal of this part of the season had been to improve 5-minute power, it was really unsuccessful. Alternatively, if you look out around 20 minutes, you can see a substantial difference between the curves, around 50 watts! Thus, if the goal here was to improve sustained power or general fitness we can say the training program has been extremely successful.

Compare this to the following graph, which is from an age group athlete who has moved beyond general fitness training to more focused work (Figure 7-5).

This is a nice example of what might be termed the "raise the left, fill the right" approach. Early in the season, the athlete worked at raising power across all durations but particularly the short durations in an effort to raise VO2max. Then, he proceeded to increase the length of time he could maintain power, during longer, more race specific efforts. Note that while there was a general rise

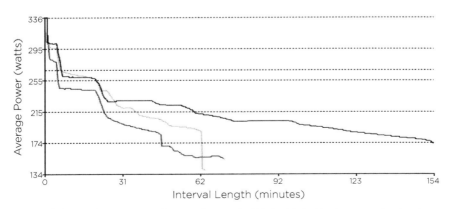

Figure 7-5. Maximum power in an advanced athlete. Note the increase in short term power, which is later followed by increases in long-term power.

in short term power from the dark gray line to the light gray line (note the 5-minute and 20-minute power output, marked by the first flattening of the line and the second flattening of the line), there is no major difference between the dark gray and the light gray except the ability to maintain power.

The point I am trying to get across to you is that analysis like this can bring your training to a totally new place. You can now know with absolute certainty if your training program is working or not. You can try different training protocols, and see if the expected improvements happen. If you don't see the expected improvements, you need to ask yourself why that might be and make the appropriate adjustments.

Using a maximal power graph like this, we can make some other important decisions and analyses. For instance, in Figure 7-5, we can see that the athlete's best performance for an hour is about 215W or so. Thus, we can immediately tell that it would be ill advised to try a 40K / 1-hour time trial at 240 watts. The curve allows you to guess at reasonable targets for workouts or races of different distances. A good rule of thumb is that you may not be able to hold a power output that is significantly higher than your recent best for that duration.

Step 3: In-depth analysis

The final step is really getting in there and looking over individual files in detail. Are you really doing what you think you are doing? For instance, are your threshold / CP intervals really threshold intervals? If not, what do you need to do to remedy the situation? Let's start out with another age group athlete who is doing 20-minute intervals at Critical Power on short rest.

What are we seeing here? The prescribed workout was 3 x 20 minutes at Critical Power with 5-minutes rest between. (Yeah, this is a really hard workout.) What we see here is a drop in power from the first, to the second to the third interval (Figure 7-6).

CHAPTER 7
The Nuts and Bolts: Rationally Analyzing Your Training

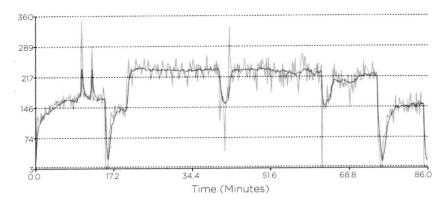

Figure 7-6. Threshold workout where the athlete attempted 3 x 20 minutes at CP. Note the failure during the 3rd interval. The athlete had not been sleeping well.

The athlete makes an effort to rescue the 3rd one, but it is a bit too little, too late. Also, look at the recovery interval: the power falls there as well. So, the athlete did not complete the workout. The important question is *why*? Was the weather unusually hot? Did the athlete do an especially hard workout earlier in the day, or the day before? Is the athlete eating enough (Table 7-1)?

In this particular case, I learned that the athlete had been having a particularly rough week at work, and had been having espe-

Symptom	Possible Cause	Possible Solution
Power falling from one interval to the next	Thermal stress	Acclimation Better cooling
	Hydration issues	Consume more fluids
	Sleep issues	Improve rest and recovery
	Nutrition issues	Higher carbohydrate intake both during activity and regular diet
	Fatigue from previous workouts	Examine meso/microcycle of training and reorganize
	Athlete not yet fit enough to complete workout	Perform same wattage in shorter intervals, and reduce the rest week to week until athlete can complete workout

Table 7-1. Problems and Solutions in Workouts.

CHAPTER 7
The Nuts and Bolts: Rationally Analyzing Your Training

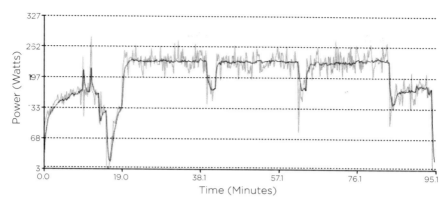

Figure 7-7. Athlete makes a successful attempt at 3 x 20 at CP.

cially poor sleep patterns. We worked out a strategy to improve rest and recovery, and a couple of days later, attempted the same workout again.

This time, he essentially nails the workout. The power still falls slightly, but we expect this will improve as he adapts to the new training load (Figure 7-7).

Of course, this begs the question, "How can I tell how much of a decrease is too much?" It's a good question, and there is no hard and fast rule. Personally, I like to go by percentage. If the power drops by more than 5% from interval to interval, or 5% within the session, I go looking for a reason. I have actually found this to be just a bit on the conservative side, but I feel it is better to undertrain someone a little bit than risk burning them out.

The interesting thing is that you can apply these exact same principles to your running and swimming workouts using this methodology. For instance, let's take a look at a running workout for a very good runner (Figure 7-8). This particular workout was a race simulation for a half-iron distance race in highly variable terrain. The goal of the workout was to maintain open half-marathon power / effort for the duration of the workout. For this athlete, that equates to roughly 310 watts, or about 4:40 per km / 7:30 per mile pace in flat terrain. This meant adjusting pace on the uphills so that

CHAPTER 7
The Nuts and Bolts: Rationally Analyzing Your Training

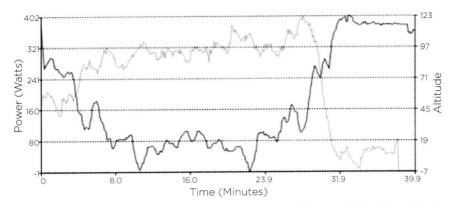

Figure 7-8. Running power output (light) and altitude (dark). Note that the athlete tries to continually advance power until failure on the final climb, where they must walk.

the athlete did not cook himself. Let's see how he fared.

We see that the athlete started out easy and then picked it up. Around 10 minutes, though, we see a problem beginning to develop. He's advanced beyond threshold power on the smaller hills, and by 25 minutes, he is pushing close to 400 watts. By about 28 minutes...pop. He's done, and has to walk to the top of the big climb. When asked about this later, we found that he was trying to maintain pace rather than effort / power.

The answer was relatively straightforward. Using RaceDay, we calculated the equivalent pace for the climb that corresponded to threshold power, and had him run that pace instead. This gave him instant feedback, and he was able to nail this workout the next time around. After a few tries, he didn't need the GPS anymore and could do it by feel.

It is possible to apply exactly the same sort of analysis to swim data. In fact, it can be very important because the intervals athletes swim in training are often quite short and hard in comparison to how they are actually racing. We can use power analysis to make sense of the workout.

Let's use one of my athletes as an example. This is a woman who likes to go really hard. The problem with this is that triathlon is really dependent upon sustained power output, and not peak power output.

Her half-iron race pace is about 1:18/100M. The problem is that she'd rather saw her arm off than swim long intervals. So, she tends to swim short intervals, but utterly buries herself in the process (Figure 7-9 and Table 7-2).

What we see here is that her highest power output segments were also the shortest, and thus least specific to the actual demands of her race. However, we calculate her xPace at about 1:15 / 100M. Thus, we would expect that the metabolic demands of the workout might be close to those as a steady swim of similar length. Was this workout as good as swimming 400's at goal race pace with perfect form? Probably not. But, it isn't a disaster either, and some part of building training schedules is taking lemons and making lemonade when possible. Now, would this workout be a reasonable stimulus

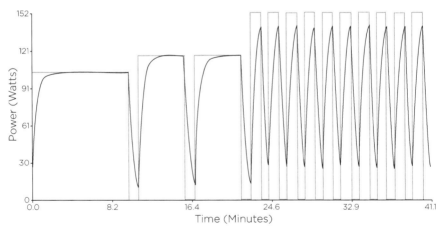

Figure 7-9. Power (light) and 25 second EWMA of power output for a swim workout.

Interval	Distance (m)	Time (min)	Time (sec)	Rest (sec)	Reps
1	800	10	11	60	1
2	400	4	56	60	2
3	100	1	8	45	10

Table 7-2. Interval Distance, Time, Rest and Repetitions.

for VO2max, since she is swimming at / above her pVO2max? Good question, and there is no clear answer. I suspect the work interval might be a little short, given that the rest interval is absolute rest, not just easier swimming.

Successful application of the principles of power-based training is about noticing both the forest and the trees, where appropriate. This becomes more and more critical as you get better and better, because gains are going to become harder to come by and you need to know where to look.

CHAPTER 8
The Dose-Response View of Training

Earlier, we talked about the idea that there is a dose-response element to training. However, what does that really mean? We talked about the dose...it's how many points you got from each workout. Now let's talk about the response and how training is absorbed and assimilated by your body, and over what period of time this new level of performance is expressed. We'll talk about this in terms of the positive and negative effects of training the body feels from each workout.

It's like this: any time an athlete trains, he or she immediately incurs both Positive Training Effect (PTE or "fitness", the dark line in Figure 8-1) and Negative Training Effect (NTE or "fatigue", the light gray line). You can think of the PTE in terms of all the good stuff that happens when you train: you are making your body get stronger and faster. You can think of the NTE in terms of the bad stuff that happens: you tear up muscle, you deplete your on-board stores of carbohydrates, that sort of thing.

The difference in increase between the PTE and NTE is specific and unique to each athlete. Everyone responds to training differently, and there are even some people who do not respond at all! The response is dependent upon factors such as genetics, and the type, volume, intensity, and frequency of training.

Using 8-1, 8-2, and 8-3, let's discuss the relationship been the Positive Training Effects and the Negative Training Effects.

Initially, the athlete's fatigue, or NTE, predominates

CHAPTER 8
The Dose-Response View of Training

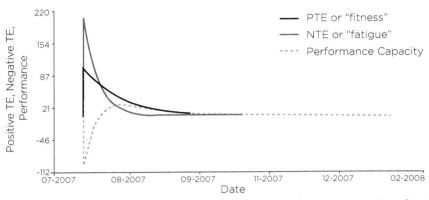

Figure 8-1. Relationship between fitness, fatigue and performance capacity after a single workout.

(Figure 8-1). Intuitively, this makes sense to us. After running a hard 10K, we know we are fitter, but we also know that we are too tired for a repeat performance. This is because our new level of fitness or PTE is masked by our fatigue. Thus, our ability to perform (dashed line) is driven down, because performance is equal to the difference between fitness and fatigue. Interestingly, the difference between how much the fitness and fatigue change with training is also specific and unique to each athlete.[34]

The next important thing to notice is that the feeling of fatigue goes away more quickly than the improved fitness; on the order of 2-5 times faster, again dependent upon the individual athlete. So, now you can see why after a few days rest you can perform better. The gray line fades, but the black line is still pretty high, so the dashed line ends up a tad higher than before. You are then able to perform better than you used to.

Now, here is the really cool part. Fitness / PTA and fatigue / NET *are additive over time* (Figure 8-2). In other words, the athlete's fitness is equal to their fitness *yesterday* (which has faded slightly) plus the new fitness gained from training *today*. The athlete's fatigue is equal to their fatigue *yesterday* (which has faded slightly) plus the new fatigue the athlete has incurred from training *today*. So, we have discovered something very interesting. Your ability to perform on any day is equal to the total of all the fitness

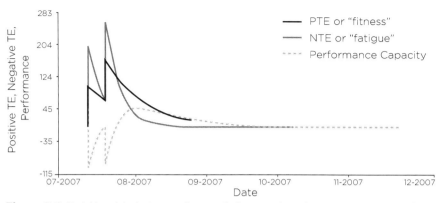

Figure 8-2. Relationship between fitness, fatigue and performance capacity after two workouts. Note the additive nature of fitness and fatigue.

and all the fatigue you ever experienced, the effect of each episode of which is slowly fading away.

Now, for the really, really cool part. If we know how fast the fatigue fades away, and we know how long the fitness hangs around, we can figure out important things. For instance, we can decide how many days of easy training we should take before trying another really hard workout. Or, we can figure out exactly how long we should taper before a big race. See, science can occasionally be useful! We'll get more into that stuff a little later on.

If you review a whole season's worth of data, you are going to see something like Figure 8-3.

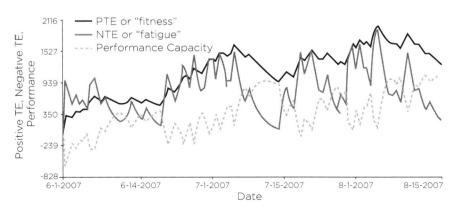

Figure 8-3. Relationship between fitness, fatigue and performance capacity over several weeks of a season. Note how performance quickly rises as fatigue falls.

CHAPTER 8
The Dose-Response View of Training

All these lines are nice, but the real question is what does it mean to you? I mean, we look at all these lines and see that they go up and down, but what does it really tell us?

Ok, first of all, remember that the vertical axis is in the units you are measuring your training in. In the above case, we can note the position of the black line in the beginning and see that this athlete absorbed about 350 BikeScore points. We also see that the gray line indicates that those 350 points of PTE "cost" the athlete 939 points of NTE. (Please remember, this relationship is different for every single athlete. This is one of the reasons I built RaceDay in the first place; to be able to figure this out on an individual basis for individual athletes). The training caused an increase in the athlete's fitness, but that investment in fitness required the athlete to accept a certain amount of fatigue. Because there was such a difference, the athlete's ability to perform (the dashed line) went down into negative territory. In other words, the athlete feels worse than when he or she started! However, as the season progresses, you can see the dashed line creeps upwards, indicating the athlete's improvement.

Now look at the period just before August of 2007. The athlete abruptly dropped the training load in order to prepare for a race, and you can see that their ability to perform shot way up! Now you can see why it is important to taper before a big race. You need rest, which drops your fatigue levels and "pays back" your fatigue balance so that you can have a great performance.

We'd like to be a bit more fancy, though. What we would like to do is figure out not just that we will feel good or bad on any given day, we want to know just how good or bad we will be, in real numbers! What you need to do is use a computer to analyze the actual performances of the athlete. It can "back calculate" what the fitness and fatigue levels must have been to result in the measured performances you have recorded. It turns out that this is pretty easy to do if you have computer software like RaceDay.

What the computer does is line up that dashed line with some of your known performances (Figure 8-4). For instance, let's say that

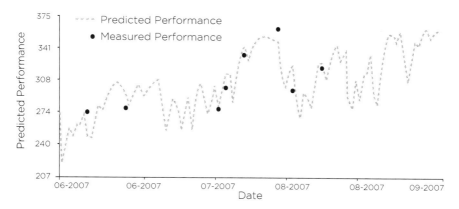

Figure 8-4. The ability of the computer to model performance. Line = prediction, black dots = measured performance. Note the high degree of correlation.

this athlete periodically tested their performance by riding a hard 3-minute interval on a loop near their house. We plot those points on top of the dashed curve, and then RaceDay adjusts how fast the fitness and fatigue rise and fall, until it gets the best match between the predictions, and the actual performance of the athlete.

Now, we have a curve that tells us exactly what we have under the hood on any given day. We can then direct future training to ensure that we are peaking on race day, or on a day when we'd like to spank our friends on a training ride, or whatever. You get the idea. By tracking this sort of data, as the song says, you can check in to see what condition your condition is in.

Perhaps more importantly, when we know just how our body is changing with training, we can make important decisions about how much and when to train in order to improve on a good schedule without risking overtraining. A great way to do this is to analyze past training logs and try to understand where things went right or wrong. Let's look at the following example, which can be found in Figure 8-5.

Take a look at the early part of the season. This athlete was building training stress over time, as evidenced by the gently climbing black line. In the beginning of February, we can see that there is a sudden spike in training load. The athlete went to a high-volume

CHAPTER 8
The Dose-Response View of Training

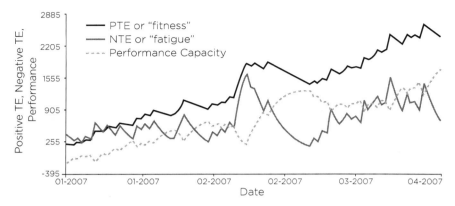

Figure 8-5. Retrospective analysis of an athlete's season. Illness occured after the large spike in training (a high-volume camp).

training camp, where a large amount of training is undertaken in a very short period of time. We can see that after this bump, there is a sudden fall off, with no training at all. The explanation is that the athlete got sick! We learned something important here. We managed to get a snapshot of what not to do again. Note the black line after the bump, it goes back to a steadier climb. Also note how the dashed line continues to climb. The athlete's fitness and performance ability are continuing to climb in a sustainable fashion.

A good rule of thumb is to ensure that once early training is established, you should try not to push the black line up by more than about 5-10% per week. This number is a bit different for different people, but this works on average and will keep you out of trouble.

Your next question is probably something like, "Can I combine scores between sports?" This is a good question. It makes intuitive sense that you ought to be able to add up points from swimming, cycling, and running to get a global idea of where your condition lies. The answer is rather complicated. For instance, we all know that riding a lot wrecks your running legs, but we don't have an idea of how much riding may help your running legs (it probably does...but just a little and in most cases only if you started out as a couch potato).

CHAPTER 8
The Dose-Response View of Training

In my first book, *Scientific Training for Triathletes,* I introduced you to the concept of specificity. Specificity means that the body adapts exactly to the stimulus applied. Some of the classic studies were done by preeminent scientists such as Dr. Ed Coyle down in Texas. What he (and innumerable others) found is that the body adapts so specifically to stress that there is very little crossover of fitness between sports.[35] For instance, Dr. Coyle demonstrated that if you take regional-class cyclists and compare them with national-class cyclists, you find that the national class guys have a higher VO2max than the regional class guys when you test them on bikes. This makes sense: national class cyclists should be able to go harder than regional class guys.

Now, the unexpected part: If you take both groups and test them on a treadmill, you find they have exactly the same VO2max. In other words, improved fitness in one sport does not cross over to another sport, even if the two sports use exactly the same body parts (legs, heart, lungs) in a very similar way.

Now, this is not true if you are looking at untrained people. If you take a couch potato, and make them ride a bike a few times a week for a couple of months, you will find they also got a little better at running. The reason for this is that you started out with a person who is so unfit that any improvement in their heart can be detected in other sports.

All this said, there was a study done on triathletes where they used the math we have been talking about and asked, "Can we find any mathematical evidence of crossover between sports?" Their results were interesting.[36] There was no evidence of crossover between swimming and anything else. There was also no crossover in fitness from running to cycling. However, there did appear to be a small crossover from cycling to running. Was it enough that we should go hunting for running gains by riding more? Almost certainly not. Should we probably be a little cautious about doing back-to-back killer bike and run sessions all the time? Almost certainly yes.

The take-home message is this: sport performance has most to do with your training in that sport. There may be a little crossover from one to another, but it is probably not enough to matter in most cases. Thus, I would argue that you should monitor each sport independently, but with the understanding that there are negative repercussions from totally shelling yourself in one sport on your performance in other sports. Put another way, it is **OK** to combine scores if you are interested in a sort of general view of how much stress you are under (i.e. "shelled" or "not shelled"). However, you should not (indeed, you cannot) expect that total sum to be useful in predicting performance in the quantitative sense.

What will be more useful to you is learning where what elite mountain bike athlete Dave Harris calls the 'pain cave' lies. In other words, if you watch the fitness and fatigue curves in the different sports, you will very quickly learn that you can predict how much of a training load (or how much of an increase in training load) you can tolerate before you start screwing up your other workouts.

Now, looking at the way these curves develop over time should give you the impression that the human body responds somewhat predictably to training. Your impression is exactly correct. In fact, once you have a model that really describes the athlete well, it is possible to perform a particular mathematical process on that model so that you can learn exactly how much effect (for better or *worse*) training on one day has on any day in the future.[37] The math is complicated, but fortunately there are tools like RaceDay that will just give you a graph that is easy to understand. Not surprisingly, it's called an Effect Curve (Figure 8-6).

You can read this Effect Curve in both directions. Let's start by reading it from left to right. The horizontal axis tells you how many days you are away from a given race, with day zero being the race day. The vertical axis tells you how much effect training on any given day has on the race on day zero, with positive numbers indicating a positive effect and negative numbers indicating a negative effect.

This should be starting to make some sense to you. You can see

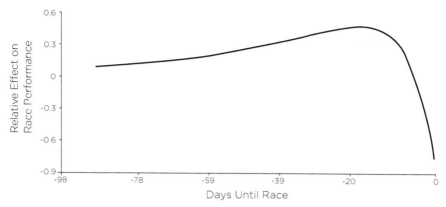

Figure 8-6. Effect of training on race performance (day zero). Note that training has a very favorable effect on race performance until a short time before the race.

that as you get closer and closer to the race, training becomes more and more important because it has more and more effect on race performance. Then, you can see a peak, and a fall off. What you are looking at is the reason you need to taper. Just before the race, recovery becomes more important. In fact, if you look at the data above, this athlete's curve drops below zero about a week before the race. That is, doing a large volume of training in the 7 days before the race will make race performance worse, not better! This is because the athlete cannot shed the fatigue in time. The best course of action is shorter, intense workouts that help maintain our training adaptations but do not contribute to the deep, lasting fatigue we get from doing a lot of training. As I mentioned in a recent interview, taper training is not about shelling yourself with more intense training than you would normally do. Rather, you want to *maintain the intensity you were already doing*.[38] In other words, keep the LT workout (maybe do more multiples with shorter work duration), and cut the long ride and run down exponentially.

All this said, it is important not to take the curve too literally. In other words, the Effect Curve is a mathematical approximation of what is going on with the athlete, not the other way around. If you took the model 100% literally, you should get the best results by not doing any training *at all* once the Effect Curve fell below the zero line, and we know from experimental evidence that this is *not true*. Thus, it is important to use models to inform your training process, however, you must understand that they are just one (very useful) tool in the greater athletic toolbox. You should not be a slave to them.

In using the Effect Curve, I have had the best results with athletes shooting for a single great performance (i.e. Kona) by starting an exponential taper at the peak of the curve and ensuring the training load has fallen substantially by the time the curve falls

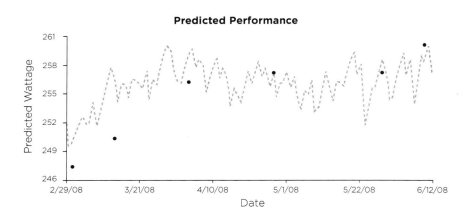

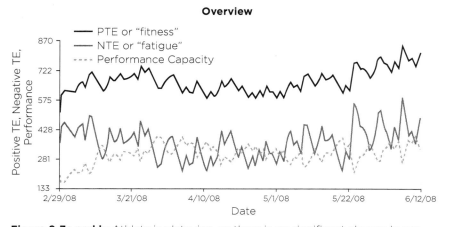

Figure 8-7a and b: Athlete is plateuing, as there is no significant change in predicted (dashed) or actual (black dots) performance in the month of May. Training is changed, leading to an increased training load (dark line) and performance capacity begins to increase again.

below the zero line. On the other hand, for athletes who a training for multiple races in a short period, I may maintain a higher load until the day the curve falls below zero, and then cut back sharply in preparation to race.

Now, as I mentioned earlier, you can read the Effect Curve in the opposite direction. That is, if we pretend day zero is a training day, and read from right to left, what we see is how long it takes to feel the benefits of that workout (when the curve crosses the zero line). We can also see how long it is until we see the maximum benefit from that workout (the peak of the curve), and how much benefit we retain as time goes on (the downward sloping portion after the peak). Now you can understand why you feel wrecked after a hard workout, but better and stronger a week or more later…it takes that long for your body to recover from, and adapt to the training load you imposed!

The most important idea I want to convey to you is that all of these fancy pictures are very different for different athletes. The fact of the matter is that the only way you can really know what is going on with an athlete is by training them hard and keeping careful track of that training, and testing performance to find out the relationship between training and performance for that athlete. We can make certain generalizations, for instance, on average many people will adapt to a given training load within 4-6 weeks. Fitness and performance will begin to plateau, and then training must be increased to continue to see improvements (Figure 8-7a and b). However, if we want to be more specific, we really need to use some of the aforementioned math to optimize our training, understand just how our bodies are responding, and then make the needed changes to continue to improve.

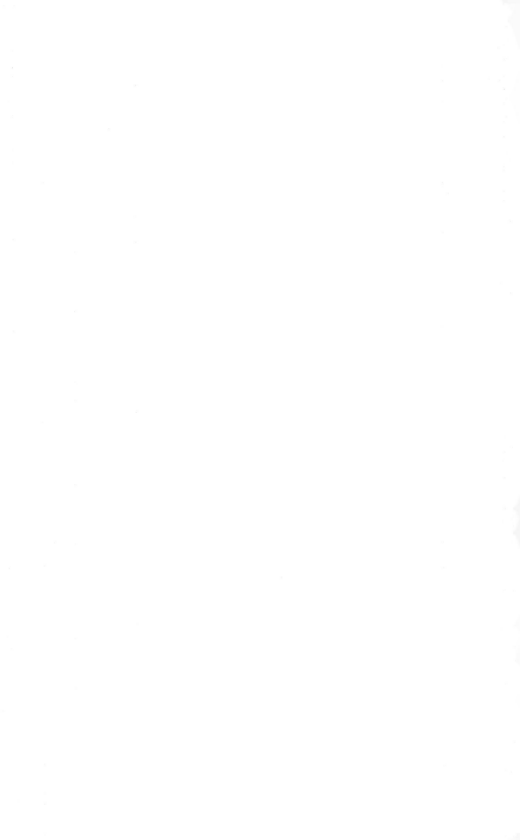

CHAPTER 9
Intelligently Planning Your Training Season, Schedule, and Workout

Ok, we now know how to benchmark our training in terms of it's relationship to Critical Power or Critical Velocity, and we also know how to set up zones based upon Critical Power or Critical Velocity in order to design workouts to address different aspects of our physiology. We also now understand how the body responds to exercise, and how that changes when training becomes more or less variable. Just as importantly, we now know how to determine our personal response to exercise using a computer.

What we now need to do is address the 800-pound gorilla in the room: **How do I set up my training program based upon all of these principles?**

The first thing I am going to ask you to do is believe in something called periodization. Periodizing a schedule simply means adjusting training as the season progresses in a logical fashion. Typically, this is done by changing the amount of training undertaken, the intensity at which you train, and the particular skills focused upon. Although Tudor Bompa is often credited as being the father of this theory, it was first formalized by L.P. Matveyev, a Russian scientist. It is worth understanding where Matveyev's theories came from, as well as the criticisms of those theories, because his approach (for better or worse) has been a major force in popular triathlon training, particularly in the United States.

It is important to understand that Matveyev did not really develop his system through an experimental approach. Rather, he looked at the preparation of Russian athletes before the 1952 Helsinki Olympics by having the athletes fill out questionnaires.[39,40] His review seemed to indicate a highly reciprocal relationship between volume and intensity, with large swings in both throughout the year.

The problem here is obvious: the whole system based upon training that happened to work for certain athletes in particular sports in the 1950's. It isn't actually based on a current understanding of exercise physiology. This said, Matveyev made the important contribution to training theory that there must be some interplay between intensity and duration of training, however, he falls flat in that he failed to address the observations of his contemporaries who believed more in the processes of biological adaptation and less in Matveyev's pedagogy. Matveyev seems to view athletic form as something that is "taught" to the athlete's body, in the same way that a student learns addition and subtraction before learning multiplication and division. In fact, the evidence-based principles of exercise physiology dictate that the body adapts to specific stress, and thus training needs to be about providing that stress in a rational way to allow adaptation and progression. Even in the early 1990's, Matveyev still urged caution in basing training theory on the "newly found" principles of biology![41]

Confusion has reigned ever since, as many authors, coaches and athletes have taken what Matveyev said too literally, often without reviewing the very valid criticisms of both his contemporaries and those who came later. In point of fact, although many popular literature books, websites, and coaches spew these teachings as though they are gospel, a quick chat with anyone actually working in elite / Olympic sport will make you realize that few athletes or coaches actually periodize their training schedules in that way, especially outside the United States. What we need is a better way to think about training.

With that in mind, let's discuss the work of the sports scientists who have come to challenge Matveyev's ideas. Tschiene, a German sports scientist, felt that this model was not applicable to top athletes, though it might work reasonably well for beginners. (I would agree with this assessment, as many amateur triathletes looking for a good race or two get decent results with a Matveyev-esque approach.) Tschiene's variation on the theme was a more microcyclic approach; that is, the athlete is always addressing volume and intensity (including year round speed work) in a significant way to establish "a very high and stable performance level" with perhaps a more subtle drop in volume and maintenance of intensity as the athlete enters the main competitive season.[42] This approach can inform our approach to triathlon provided that we understand intensity to mean *race specific* intensity. In other words, you don't need to shell long-course athletes with epic VO2max training three times a week. I have found the "raise and hold" aspect of Tschiene's theory extremely effective for professional athletes with long racing seasons. I also agree with his support of the principles of Mellenberg, Saidchusin and Verkhoshansky (see below), who suggested the need to use frequent field testing to monitor how closely the athlete's performance status approaches the requirements of competition.

The most stinging criticism of the blind application of Matveyev's doctrine comes from Verkhoshansky, who attempts to use principles of physiology as the basis of proper periodization.[43, 44, 45] Although his work is too far reaching to review extensively here, I will attempt to distill the salient points for triathlon training. Essentially, Professor Verkhoshanky postulates that athletes have two "gears": one is below threshold power, which is run on the basis of the slow-twitch muscle fibers and oxidative metabolism, and the other is "above threshold", which is heavily reliant upon the fast-twitch fibers, glycolyisis and creatine phosphate. He advocates that the best way to train, then, is prolonged efforts at threshold effort to effectively "raise the ceiling", to use the house analogy we have employed in this book. However, he also seems to believe that early speed training may lead to "cardiac dystrophy". He offers no further explanation, and I am unaware of any modern medical opinion to support his contention. It is possible he is referring to "athletic heart", which is now considered to be a normal adaptation to training by sports physicians.[46]

Verkhoshansky focuses heavily on the need for plyometric training, including "bouncy running", as well as explosive weight training. While quite useful, I believe the weight techniques he (along with Bosch and Klomp) advocates are likely better applied to athletes at the elite level, under the supervision of a highly experienced trainer, than they are to the average age-group triathlete in a local gym.

At the end of the day, there are elements that can be taken from each school of thought. If pressed, however, I would have to say that Verkhoshanky's framework and thought process is likely the one that best corresponds to physiology as we understand it, with the caveat that no system can be perfect or have all the answers.

With our little review complete, perhaps now you can see how periodization has been misunderstood to mean that your season must develop from doing high volume, low intensity training to a lesser amount of much harder work as the competitive season approaches, i.e. what amounts to the Matveyev model. However, we need to address other issues as well, as periodization has often also been misunderstood to mean you must have three progressively harder weeks per month, followed by an easier week. I'm not here to tell you that going from high volume / low intensity to low volume / high intensity is necessarily wrong, nor am I saying that the 3 "on" / 1 "off" idea must be dismissed out of hand. What I'm trying to explain is that they are both misunderstandings of what peri-

> **Periodization:** The adjustment of training as the season progresses in a logical fashion. Typically, this is done by changing the amount of training undertaken, the intensity at which you train, and the particular skills focused upon.

odization should be all about, and that no one approach is correct in every single situation. Thus, for the moment, I'd like you to forget any preconceived notions you may have about periodization, and rebuild the concept using common sense and some of the concepts I have taught you both in this book and in *Scientific Training for Triathletes*. What I want to do is teach you a thought process, rather than a specific recipe, so that you can adapt training to any athlete, at any ability level, at any distance.

There are 5 guidelines to successful periodization in triathlon. We'll tackle each in turn.

1 **Training must go from general to specific:** Early or "base" training is not about training slowly all the time. It is about addressing all aspects of fitness. As race time approaches, we then focus primarily upon what is necessary for race success.

2 **Training must be specific to the sport(s):** The scientific literature has been clear on this for about as long as there has been a field of exercise science. You need to maximize your time training for your specific sport(s), and minimize the time you spend doing other things (i.e. "cross-training" by doing a lot of time on the elliptical trainer, doing step aerobics, or playing foozball or whatever).

3 **Training must be specific to the physiological systems:** It's not enough to train by going long and slow all the time and then just hoping you can go fast in the race. You need to spend time working at, and harder than race power / pace if you expect to reach your potential.

4 **The training schedule must account for the positive and negative effects of all training:** As you learned in the last chapter there are both positive and negative effects to training. We need to be cognizant of both and realize that these effects are additive, and that we must eventually allow ourselves to recover if we want to perform at our best. We must always realize that if we are going to train three sports, we must intelligently manage how badly we fatigue ourselves in any one sport.

5 **Training must be short and fast before it is long and fast:** Early season training needs to include some amount of VO_2 work, however, this does not mean you should go out to the track and start banging out 1000M repeats at your 3K PR pace. You *will* get hurt. Start out with a few, short repeats, and then build time and number of repetitions as tolerated.

Let's try constructing a season. We will do this in a logical, step-wise fashion.

Step 1: Event Selection
Begin by selecting the correct event, and noting what is more important and what is less important, relatively speaking. Note that this does not mean MOST important and NOT important. All of the physiological systems are extremely important for every race distance. However, we cannot train the same way all the time in some sort of shotgun approach to fitness, thinking that we can maximally improve everything all at once.

Iron

Importance	Factor
More important	Fatigue Resistance
	Lactate Threshold
Less important	VO_2max

Half-Iron

Importance	Factor
More important	Lactate Threshold
	Fatigue Resistance
Less important	VO_2max

Sprint/Olympic Distance

Importance	Factor
More important	Lactate Threshold
	VO2max
Less important	Fatigue Resistance

Step 2: Season Construction / Building The Macrocycle

First, commit the Macrocycle Schema to memory. It is useful for racing at any distance (Figure 9-1).

In every case, our goal is to move from general to very specific (that is, race specific) fitness. Our progression is always moving towards doing exactly what we need to do, exactly as hard as (or even a little harder than) we need to be doing it. If you are planning on riding an iron-distance bike leg at 220 watts, you'd best have done many long intervals at that power, and then spend some time running off the bike after riding that hard to be sure you can do it.

Let's look at some specific schema for different race distances. The exact length of the periods can be anywhere from 4-8 weeks, with 6 weeks representing a reasonable medium. This is, on average, how long the body takes to adapt to any new training load. This can be "tweaked" using the data from the impulse response models, or by carefully watching the athlete's performance ability.

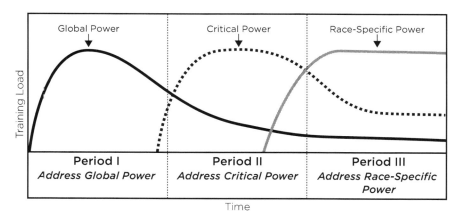

Figure 9-1. Distribution of power / pace training over the course of the season. Exact transitions between periods is dependent on individual athlete needs and background.

CHAPTER 9
Intelligently Planning Your Training Season, Schedule, and Workout

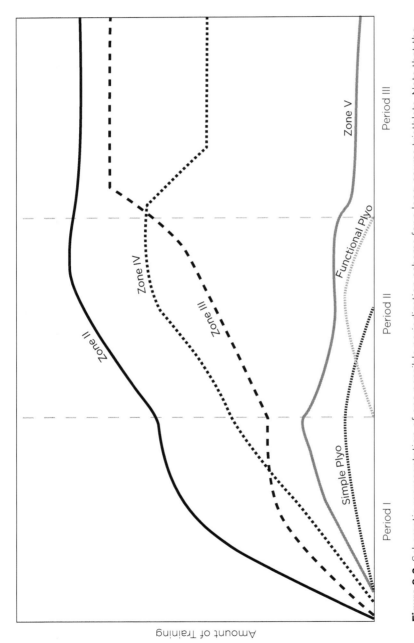

Figure 9-2. Schematic representation of one possible periodization scheme for a long-course triathlete. Note that the optimal strategy will be different for every different athlete, based upon their personal strengths, weaknesses, background and event selection.

After a plateau in performance for a week or two, it is likely safe to advance the program, either by increasing the training load, changing the mix of intensity and duration of training, or moving to the next period. You make the decision based upon how much time you have before competition, and what you can reasonably hope to accomplish in that time frame. (Do not *increase* the training if the athlete's performances are *decreasing*. We'll discuss the reasons for that later.)

Period I focuses on a broad treatment of fitness: sport specific strength, speed, and endurance. The main goal here is preparation for the more specific training to come. Period II focuses very specifically on limiters to performance, including a careful focus on the physiological systems most critical for race performance. Period III continues that focus on the physiological limiters, but does it in a manner that more closely matches the specific demands of the race. For instance, were we training an iron-distance athlete, it would be possible to address Critical Power / threshold power on the bike through one or more weekly workouts that included 2 x 20 minute efforts at threshold power. These would be appropriate for Period II, but would morph as we enter Period III. We would select longer intervals in the high tempo range perhaps 4 x 30 minutes, since that is where our athlete will race.

Step 3: Build The Periods

This is the point were we begin to get a bit more specific. In this case, we'll consider a hypothetical, high level age group athlete. Let's consider Period I, where we want to address fitness broadly.

Period I:

Period I has a general focus. The black line indicates the build in endurance (Zone II) training, which is critical to help build fatigue resistance. The dotted line indicates threshold stimulus, which is critical to improve metabolic fitness. The gray line indicates VO_2 (Zone V) stimulus, which increases aerobic capacity, primarily through improving the maximal pumping capacity of the heart. This is delayed slightly with respect to the other zones, primarily because of the stress and injury risk of the training, and because the process of cardiac adaptation is begun with other training.

Plyometrics are key in improving running economy, primarily through stiffening the soft tissues of the body and permitting more elastic rebound. As we discussed earlier, it is thought that this occurs via improved reflex arcs that can help pretension the muscles before footstrike. These exercises begin during this period and gently increase. Up front, these are short box jumps or hurdle hops. Later, they evolve into functional bounding and more complex exercises, such as those suggested by Verkhoshansky, Bosch and Klomp (see Chapter 3 for details).

Period II:

Period II sees the focus begin the changeover from general to specific. Endurance training and threshold training begin to climb. Metabolic fitness is addressed specifically by hard threshold training: intervals at 100% of Critical Power. Our aim is to build training load towards the limit the athlete is capable of tolerating. By the end of this cycle, the athlete will have built substantial fatigue. It is critical to manage this fatigue effectively through proper nutrition and sleep, and judicious use of recovery workouts. We see a decrease in VO2 training to a maintenance level, and a decrease in simple plyometrics. The drop in simple plyometrics will be more than made up for by the small amount of functional plyometrics, and the increase in running volume.

By the end of Period II, the athlete should be capable of completing the goal event. They should not necessarily be able to have a peak performance, however, they should have banked enough training such that they could successfully participate without complete fatigue or injury. If the coach (or athlete) determines that this is not the case, the athlete should not proceed to Period III, but address any perceived problems.

Period III:

Period III is focused on the specific demands of the race. For half-iron and iron-distance athletes, there is a stabilization of endurance training, and a stabilization / decrease in absolute threshold training. That "pure" threshold stimulus is replaced and compensated for by increases in tempo / race pace specific training. VO_2 training is decreased to a lower level, and plyometric exercises are eliminated. In contrast, sprint and Olympic-distance athletes would see a relatively larger decrease in long endurance training, a continued push towards threshold work, including weekly or biweekly bricks, and possibly a slight build in VO_2 work, depending on race terrain and/or format.

In any case, the period usually ends with a taper, decreasing duration more than intensity, in preparation to race. However, this is not a hard a fast rule. The question of what to do with regard to tapering can be difficult. If the athlete is racing frequently and/or has a long season ahead, tapering must necessarily be limited, otherwise the athlete will be constantly tapering rather than training. In those cases, it is often most beneficial to bring the training up to a high level, allow the performance status of the athlete to rise as well, and then simply maintain the overall training load with brief periods of recovery in the days before the races (i.e. a "mini-taper" that occurs during the days the Effect Curve falls below zero, see page 79 for more on this).

When we speak about decreasing volume more than intensity, it is important that we have a clear idea about what we mean to do. As we discussed earlier, tapering is not about cutting your training hours by two-thirds and then flogging yourself with all-out 400's on the track. Rather, it is about the smart application of specific intensity. In other words, while tapering for a half-iron distance race, we may reduce total training load (i.e. BikeScore) on the bike by about half through an exponential reduction in endurance training. However, we would maintain intensity by continuing the LT stimulus through maintaining our Zone IV sessions during the week before the race. This allows us to freshen up while ensuring that we maintain all of those hard-won metabolic adaptations. We might also include some low-stress VO2 work (perhaps a few 30/30 type intervals) or strides to keep ourselves feeling sharp.

The Place of Recovery in Period Construction

There are conflicting schools of thought on recovery. The first is that recovery periods must be scheduled at regular intervals (i.e. the 3 weeks "on" / 1 week "off" plan so common with amateur triathletes and other endurance athletes in the U.S.). The other is that recovery should be taken when it is needed and the amount adjusted on the fly. This strategy seems to be a bit more common in elite sport where athletes are closely monitored.

There isn't a consensus agreement on this. However, two things remain clear. First, there is **no** physiological reason anyone must have 3 weeks "on" and one week "off". Secondly, racheting up the volume constantly will result in problems.[47] Both training stimulus and recovery time must be carefully adjusted over time to ensure the optimal results. I wish there was a recipe, but there isn't. You need to learn to listen to your body, or teach your athlete to listen to theirs if you are a coach. This is important enough that we will discuss in the segment on recovery at the end of this chapter.

Step 4: Constructing and Developing the Key Workouts Of the Period

The next step is to develop the key workout for the period in the context of each microcycle / week. It is important not to over-think this. In point of fact, there is no reason a microcycle should be 7 days long. It could be 8 days or 10 days or 14 days. All this said, athletes tend to understand schedules better when they work on a time course they are familiar with, and tend to follow them when they fit in with the other predictable events in their lives, i.e. work schedules on weekdays and family/personal commitments on the weekends. For the sake of argument, we'll work with weeks in this section. We will also assume we are working with an athlete who has maintained some training through a couple of workouts in each sport during the off season, and hasn't become a total couch potato.

Period I:

Endurance and Tempo Workouts: Endurance and tempo workouts can be written into the same session, with the amount of each varied appropriately. Typically, volume should be advanced ahead of intensity in this particular workout, but this is not a hard and fast rule. For instance, in the case of an average age group athlete who wants to race at the half-iron or iron distance, a weekly long, endurance paced ride might be stretched to 3 hours, and then 10 minute intervals at tempo power would be introduced. We first increase the number of repetitions, and then decrease the rest. The progression might be:

Bike Scheme

Week 1:	2.5 hours in Zone II
Week 2:	3 hours in Zone II with 2 x 10 minutes in Zone III with 5 minutes recovery
Week 3:	3 hours in Zone II with 4 x 10 minutes in Zone III with 5 minutes recovery
Week 4:	3.5 hours in Zone II with 4 x 10 minutes in Zone III on 2.5 minutes recovery
Week 5:	3.5 hours in Zone II with 2 x 20 minutes in Zone III on 5 minutes recovery
Week 6:	4 hours in Zone II with 2 x 20 minutes in Zone III on 5 minutes recovery

The progression for running will be similar, but with fewer hours / miles. Typically, I don't like to stretch the long run beyond 75 minutes in Period I for age group athletes, and will often settle for less, particularly if the athlete has not been running much in the off season.

Run Scheme

Week 1:	40 minutes in Zone II
Week 2:	45 minutes in Zone II with 1 x 5 minutes in Zone III on 5 minutes recovery
Week 3:	50 minutes in Zone II with 2 x 5 minutes in Zone III on 5 minutes recovery
Week 4:	45 minutes in Zone II with 3 x 5 minutes in Zone III on 5 minutes recovery
Week 5:	55 minutes in Zone II with 4 x 5 minutes in Zone III on 5 minutes recovery
Week 6:	60 minutes in Zone II with 2 x 10 minutes in Zone III on 5 minutes recovery

The above goals for cycling and running would not be wildly different between race distances, with the possible exception of sprint triathlon, where you can probably safely give up some saddle time, unless you are really trying to race at the pointy end of the field.

Swimming workouts are usually built a bit differently and more creatively. Since swimming form is so critical, and since swimmers lose form as they tire, we cannot be as metricratic in our approach to it. Or rather, we can try, but the focus needs to be on quality swimming with good form. Each workout must always come with the caveat, "Bag the workout if you feel your form start to break down."

Barring changes in form, you can construct a similar progression. Early in the period, endurance intervals should begin in chunks of 300M, and stretch to 500-600M by the end of the period. Rather than changing pace mid-interval, however, I usually break out the tempo-paced intervals. I start them out at 200M and may stretch to 400 by the end of Period I.

Threshold Workouts: The threshold workouts should be carried out in a low stress context to begin with. As intimated earlier in the book, this could be written as multiples of 5-minute intervals at threshold power or pace, with intermediate rest intervals shortened until the athlete arrives at 2 x 15-20 minutes at threshold power with 2-5 minutes rest between.

Bike Scheme

Week 1:	1 hours in Zone II with 4 x 5 minutes in Zone IV with 5 minutes recovery
Week 2:	1.25 hours in Zone II with 4 x 5 minutes in Zone IV with 2.5 minutes recovery
Week 3:	1.5 hours in Zone II with 2 x 10 minutes in Zone IV with 5 minutes recovery
Week 4:	1.5 hours in Zone II with 2 x 10 minutes in Zone IV on 2.5 minutes recovery
Week 5:	1.5 hours in Zone II with 2 x 15 minutes in Zone IV on 5 minutes recovery
Week 6:	1.5 hours in Zone II with 2 x 15 minutes in Zone IV on 2.5 minutes recovery

I would write these workouts irrespective of the race distance. Threshold power development is critical at every race distance and always needs to be addressed.

Because of the increased risk of injury, threshold running needs to be added in a much more judicious manner. In Period I, the total workout length might be only 45 minutes or so. We do the threshold running on a track or measured course to closely monitor and adjust the amount of work done. Typically, I may begin Period I with 4 x 400M at threshold pace / Zone IV on equal rest intervals (i.e. 400M easy jog), and build to 7 or 8 repeats by the end of the period. A good, specific pace target is open 10K pace in the absence of good Critical Velocity data.

Threshold stimulus may be inserted into swim workouts as 100-200M intervals to begin with. The exact length and number of repeats must again be adjusted to the skill of the swimmer. Threshold swimming needs to be smooth and directed. If you or your athlete is barely hitting the splits, thrashing furiously in the water, the solution is usually not more swimming, but addressing issues of form.

VO2 Workouts: Because of the stressful nature of these workouts, they need to start out short and sweet. A nice way of starting off is with the "30/30" workouts popularized by Dr. Veronique Billat, which we discussed earlier. Basically, these workouts involve executing 30 seconds at VO2 / Level V power or pace, then 30 seconds of recovery, repeated many times over. Because the intervals are short, the chance of injury is low, and the athlete or coach is able to easily terminate the workout if form becomes an issue. It is possible to ballpark this as 3K pace if test data is unavailable.

By the end of Period I, the work interval may be extended to several repeats of 2-3 minutes with equal rest. On the track, this may be done as 400M-800M repeats, and in the pool as 100-200M repeats.

Simple Plyometric Workouts: We can begin here with the box jumps, hurdle hops, and combinations of the two (Chapter 3). These are typically relatively safe and easily mastered, and can be built without too much fear of overload. Doing more than 20 minutes or so of this type of work, 3-4 times a week is likely more than enough.

Functional Plyometric Workouts: N/A

Period II:

Endurance and Tempo Workouts: Moving into Period II, we must start prioritizing workouts and begin the process of differentiating training based upon race distance. We must ensure that we can cover the race distance in a reasonable time frame. This requires fatigue resistance, and the most specific way to address this is by lifting the time spent training. However, our goal is not simply to flog ourselves with insane volumes of training. Our training should at some point approach race time, particularly on the bike, but there must again be periods of directed work which I usually apply as tempo riding. For an iron or half-iron distance athlete, I might write a progression as follows.

Bike Scheme

Week 1:	4 hours in Zone II with 2 x 20 minutes in Zone III on 5 minutes recovery
Week 2:	4 hours in Zone II with 2 x 20 minutes in Zone III on 5 minutes recovery
Week 3:	4.5 hours in Zone II with 5 x 10 minutes in Zone III with 5 minutes recovery
Week 4:	5 hours in Zone II with 5 x 10 minutes in Zone III on 2.5 minutes recovery
Week 5:	6 hours in Zone II with 3 x 20 minutes in Zone III on 5 minutes recovery
Week 6:	5 hours in Zone II with 3 x 20 minutes in Zone III on 5 minutes recovery

For sprint and Olympic distance athletes, I would typically cap the long / endurance riding at 3 hours or so, again depending upon the quality and level of the athlete. High level age groupers and pros can still benefit from 3-4 hour long rides.

Again, it is important to be careful with running. Though the athlete will be on the run course for anywhere from 2.75 to 4.5 hours in the iron-distance realm, and since it just isn't feasible to do that kind of running in training, we are beholden to leaning more towards manipulating the intensity / frequency than we are the distance. Thus, even though distance will peak during this period, I keep the long run to a limit of about 90-100 minutes in amateurs and no longer than about 2 hours in elites / professionals.

Run Scheme

Week 1:	50 minutes in Zone II
Week 2:	60 minutes in Zone II with 4 x 5 minutes in Zone III on 5 minutes recovery

Week 3:	70 minutes in Zone II with 2 x 10 minutes in Zone III on 5 minutes recovery
Week 4:	80 minutes in Zone II with 2 x 15 minutes in Zone III on 5 minutes recovery
Week 5:	90 minutes in Zone II with 2 x 20 minutes in Zone III on 5 minutes recovery
Week 6:	90 minutes in Zone II with 5 x 10 minutes in Zone III on 5 minutes recovery

At the sprint and Olympic distances, we might limit the long run to around 75 minutes, however, there is no harm and probably some benefit in pushing the higher level age groupers and elites to 90 minutes.

Swimming should include a long workout at this point, often including 500-800M intervals on short rest, with at least some segment of it devoted to race pace / tempo or faster swimming. Again, monitoring of form is critical, and hopefully this was addressed in detail during Period I. Here, we are no longer trying to make major changes in form. While some drills are appropriate, at some point it is necessary to "play the hand we are dealt", so to speak.

Threshold Workouts: During Period II, our primary focus is on stressing power / pace at LT. These workouts are relatively short with respect to the eventual race distance, and are also quite taxing. By the end of the period, there should likely be a second workout per week that includes this sort of work. Dietary carbohydrates should be closely monitored; this is no time to be surviving on salad and water.

Bike Scheme

Week 1:	1.5 hours in Zone II with 2 x 15 minutes in Zone IV on 2.5 minutes recovery
Week 2:	1.5 hours in Zone II with 2 x 20 minutes in Zone IV with 2.5 minutes recovery

Week 3:	1.5 hours in Zone II with 5 x 10 minutes in Zone IV with 5 minutes recovery
Week 4:	2 x 1.5 hour workouts. One includes 2 x 20 in Zone IV, one includes 2 x 10 in Zone IV
Week 5:	2 x 1.5 hour workouts. One includes 2 x 20 in Zone IV, one includes 3 x 10 in Zone IV
Week 6:	2 x 1.5 hour workouts. One includes 2 x 20 in Zone IV, one includes 4 x 10 in Zone IV

In short course athletes at the amateur level, it is often possible to get by with a single 2 x 20 workout per week / microcycle. Again, we adjust this to the level of the athlete. Better athletes need more than less experienced athletes.

We advance the threshold work in running as well. In Period I, the total workout length was only 45 minutes or so, but we build this to an hour or more in Period II, depending upon the level and ability of the athlete. Again, we do all threshold running on a track or marked course to closely monitor the amount of work done. Typically, I begin Period I with 3 x 800M at Threshold Pace / Zone IV on equal rest intervals (i.e. 800M easy jog), and build to 5-8 repeats by the end of the period, depending upon the level of the athlete. The interval may be stretched to 1K in elite / professional athletes. We focus closely on even splitting; when pace starts to fall off, it is time to bag the workout.

VO2 Workouts: At this point, power / pace at VO_2 has been well established, and the goal is no longer great improvement, but maintenance. Depending upon the level of the athlete, and how threshold power develops, it can become necessary to return to this type of work. (Recall the earlier discussion using the analogy of the house, and what to do if you are having problems "raising the ceiling." See page 21 for details.)

Simple Plyometric Workouts: At this point, we begin the move from simple to functional plyometric workouts.

Functional Plyometric Workouts: Functional plyometrics involve running and bounding. Again, these sorts of workouts are the icing on the cake at 15 to 20 minutes, 3 times weekly. We wrap these up before the end of the cycle again and do not revisit them, as we will have bigger fish to fry (i.e. more specific work to do) as the race approaches.

Period III:

Endurance And Tempo Workouts: During Period III, we settle into the most race-specific training we can, without neglecting the other important aspects of fitness. For iron and half-iron distance racing, we maintain a long ride with a larger proportion of it occupied by very race specific power output. During this period, it is important to either do some race simulations, or some brick workouts where the athlete runs off the bike 30-60 minutes with some 10-20 minute intervals at goal race pace. If the athlete can easily even split the efforts, chances are that he or she will be able to run similarly during the race. If it is a struggle, it is time to reevaluate the goal race power / pace on the bike and / or run.

Bike Scheme

Week 1:	5 hours in Zone II with 3 x 20 minutes in Zone III on 5 minutes recovery (+ Brick Run 30 min)
Week 2:	5 hours in Zone II with 4 x 20 minutes in Zone III on 5 minutes recovery (+ Brick Run 30 min)
Week 3:	5 hours in Zone II with 3 x 30 minutes in Zone III with 5 minutes recovery (+ Brick Run 40 min)
Week 4:	4.5 hours in Zone II with 4 x 30 minutes in Zone III on 2.5 minutes recovery (+ Brick Run 45 min)
Week 5:	4.5 hours in Zone II with 4 x 30 minutes in Zone III on 5 minutes recovery (+ Brick Run 50 min)
Week 6:	4.5 hours in Zone II with 4 x 30 minutes in Zone III on 5 minutes recovery (+ Brick Run 50 min)

For short course racing, the "long" ride can be cut back to approximately 2.5 hours, which should be more than 50% dedicated to tempo riding. Essentially, this ride becomes an exercise in pushing up power / pace at lactate threshold from below, while the threshold ride becomes an exercise in pulling it up from above. It should also occasionally end in a brick run.

Running can sometimes be tough to manage during this period of time. For elites racing the iron distance, it would not be unusual to push the long run to 2 hours in the early part of Period III before cutting it back and making the run a fair bit harder in terms of intensity. Only the best age groupers should be going that long and then only rarely. The recovery costs are simply too high.

Threshold Workouts: During this time period, the threshold stimulus moves back to a maintenance 2 x 20 minute interval workout for the long course athletes. Most of what you need will be coming from the extensive amount of tempo work during the long ride.

On the run, because there is a limit to how long most athletes can go, it is often advisable to slightly delay backing off of the 800M-1K intervals, usually until the second week of the cycle. At this point, we then rely more on the longer tempo intervals to make up for the loss of pure LT stimulus.

We need to do something a bit different for short course racing, since we will be racing it so much harder. Here, we are making up for our loss of volume on the long days with an increase in intensity. I like to do this by including a hard trainer / track session, where after a warm up the athlete will ride for 10 minutes at critical power, and run 1000-1600M at goal race pace / 10K pace (or even a few seconds faster), repeated several times. I include this in addition to the usual threshold workout.

VO2 Workouts: During Period III, the least important element is VO2max work, at least as far as the iron and half-iron distance athletes are concerned. Note I did not say 'unimportant'. It still needs to be there, just in a less dramatic form. It doesn't take much to maintain a set of 100M intervals in the pool or 400's on the track. I usually move the bike stimulus into a weekly set of 4 x 2 minutes at VO2max with equal rest.

For the short course racers, the application of VO2max training is dependent upon the race format / terrain. For instance, if there are lots of short, steep climbs, this type of training needs to be included in some significant way. If the athlete is racing ITU / draft legal, then it is extremely important as well. I cannot overemphasize just how specific training must be to the demands of the particular type of racing the athlete is going to be doing.

Simple Plyometric Workouts: N/A

Functional Plyometric Workouts: N/A

Step 5: Arranging the Key Workouts Within The Microcycle / Week

Unfortunately, the arrangement of workouts within a microcycle is often problematic. The process need not be overly thought out or micro-managed. The most important thing to remember is that the hard workouts need to be hard and/or long, and the easy workouts need to be easy. As we'll discuss later, the best way to overtrain someone is not to make their hard workouts harder, but to make their easy workouts harder.

I usually begin building the week by placing the weekly long workouts where they need to be based upon the athlete's schedule. If the athlete needs to do all the long stuff on the weekend (not uncommon for many people), that is the way it is going to have to be. If the athlete is a great cyclist and a relatively weaker runner, I usually write in the run on the Saturday and the bike / brick on the Sunday. The long swim can go on either day (in Period III, this becomes a race specific swim). If the opposite is true, the run and ride are reversed. In either case, Monday becomes a recovery day that is either entirely off, or maybe with a little easy swimming. For age groupers, a day off for the sake of sanity is often a prerequisite for a happy athlete.

I then try to alternate the threshold sessions and VO2 sessions in the middle of the week. The threshold sessions are often quite taxing, and require a fair bit of recovery, whereas the VO2 sessions feel pretty hard at the time, but generally do not require the same amount of recovery unless you fry yourself. Again, you should be finishing these feeling like you still had a couple left in you. Thus, the short, hard stuff gives the muscles a breather from the long, sustained and ultimately more fatiguing threshold workouts.

I am always hesitant to actually provide a schedule, because doing so means I run the risk of people blindly applying it as though it was the best thing for every athlete, always. Thus, the following week represents a sample cycle from Period III for a typical age-group / middle-of-the-pack athlete racing at the half-iron distance. It merely represents one possible way, and not the only way, of doing things. The appropriate training for you or anyone else might be substantially different.

The place of recovery in microcycle scheduling

Above, we discussed the idea of recovery in the context of the periods, in other words, when to schedule a period of "down time" to allow regeneration and compensation for the damage caused by training. In my opinion, it is possible that regeneration is of more importance in the context of the weekly schedule.

Power training in the way I present it in this book is not easy. I have seen how it effects athletes, and I have felt how it affects me personally. It is remarkably easy to push an athlete over the edge by constantly trying to lift training stress. With this in mind, a good place to begin is with a weekly day off. It gives the mind and body a break. It allows you to catch up on your nutrition and be sure that the muscles have been maximally repleted with glycogen for the next round of training. It gives you a chance to think about

CHAPTER 9
Intelligently Planning Your Training Season, Schedule, and Workout

	Monday	Tuesday	Wednesday	Thursday	Friday	Saturday	Sunday
SESSION I	OFF	**LT ride:** 20 min endurance ride @ 160W. **Main set:** 2x 20 minutes at 230 watts with 5 min recovery @ 150W between. 20 min endurance ride @ 160W	**Endurance run with VO2 intervals:** 15 minutes @ 8:30 / mile pace **Main set:** On marked course or track: 5 x 400 @ 1:36 / 400, 400 easy recover. 15 minutes @ 8:30 / mile pace	**LT run:** 15 min @ 8:30 / mile pace **Main set:** 3 x 1 mile @ 6:50 /mile pace with 5 minutes easy jog recovery. 15 min @ 8:25 / mile pace	**Endurance ride with VO2 intervals:** Total ride is 1.5 hours endurance riding at 160 Watts **Main set:** 5 x 2 minutes at 280W, 2 min easy recover between.	**Long ride:** 4 hours endurance riding @ 160-170W. Stay focused and maintain power throughout. **Main set:** 4 x 20 minutes tempo riding @ 200W, 5 minutes easy recovery riding between **Run off bike:** 30 minutes, build over first 15 minutes to 7:30 pace and hold.	**Long run:** 80 minutes endurance running @ 8:25 / mile pace. Include 3 x 1 mile at 7:30 / mile pace on short recovery.
SESSION II	OFF	**Endurance run with stride session:** **Run:** 60 minutes @ 8:30 / mile pace **Include:** Stride session 5 x 200 @ 45 sec / 200. Focus on quick turnover and light foot-strike		**Easy recovery ride:** 1 hour easy riding at <160 watts			
SESSION III	OFF		**VO2 swim:** Warm-up easy 500M choice 1 x 400 IM easy 3 x 300, descend from 1:50 to 1:45 / 100 by 100's, 1:30 rest **Main set:** 10 x 100 @ 1:37 / 100M on 1:00 rest Warm-up easy 500M choice		**LT swim:** Warm-up easy 500M choice 1 x 400 IM easy **Main set:** 6 x 300 @ 1:45 / 100, 2:00 rest Cool-down easy 500M choice		**Race-specific swim:** Warm-up easy 200M choice, 1 x 200 easy IM by 50's 4 x 200 @ 1:45 /100, 1:30 rest **Main set:** 4 x 500 @ 1:48 / 100, 1:30 rest. Take first 100 out hard and then settle into pace. Lengthen rest interval if you feel your form breaking down in the last 100. Cool down easy 400M choice

Table 9-1. Sample week (Period III) for a typical age group athlete racing at the half-iron distance.

everything you did in the past week and decide what could have been better or what ought to have been changed.

Must there be a day off? No. You could ride your bike to the coffee shop and call that recovery instead. However, fully addressing recovery takes more than stressing out over taking a day off or not taking a day off. It requires intelligently organizing the week so that you are not performing killer workouts day-in and day-out and running yourself into the ground.

Step 6: Follow the Plan, Evaluate the Efficacy, and Revise!

The best laid plans are useless if you don't follow them, and the most carefully followed plans are useless if they don't work for you. You owe it to yourself to know exactly what you have under the hood at any given time. This requires testing. The added benefit is that you can feed the test results into something like RaceDay to make sure your training is improving consistently. If it isn't, it is time to readdress the program and ferret out the problem. Your big race is not the time to find out that you have blown your training.

Typically, I prescribe short and long tests. This may simply be a 2-5 minute test in each sport every week to two weeks, and a monthly test that is longer (i.e. a hard 20-minute effort, or critical power / critical velocity testing). This has the added benefit of helping you adjust your training zones to ensure that you are always working at the appropriate intensity. This also allows you to plug your performance data into RaceDay and calculate your specific response to training, which will remove a lot of guesswork from the process.

If you or your athlete are really unwilling to do regular testing, you must at a minimum carefully monitor your power / pace during short and long interval workouts to ensure you are continuing to improve over time.

Final notes on recovery

Two things should be abundantly clear to you at this point. The first is that power-based training is hard. The second is that seeing major improvements in performance require allowing the body to adequately adapt to training, and that the greatest improvements come with real rest and recovery. This permits the body to shed the negative effects of training and the athlete to come to a new peak.

The $25,000 question is how to gauge the need for recovery. Too little, and it is likely that you will underperform and become overreached, or in the worst cases, overtrained. Too much, and it is likely that you will never come into your best form and will also underperform. After coaching athletes at all levels for the better part of 15 years, and working in the medical field for 10, I can tell you that you are far better off undercooking yourself by 5% than you are overcooking yourself by 1%. In the big picture, my advice is when in doubt, rest or take an easy day.

All that said, what do we really know about training / overtraining athletes? Overtraining is a complex problem. It is characterized by a somewhat nebulous collection of complaints (i.e. deep and lasting fatigue), and in some cases, measurable pathophysiologic abnormalities. It also includes what noted exercise physiologist Dr. Carl Foster has termed, "performance incompetence".[48] Now, we know from the modeling chapter that a loss of performance ability is normal until adaptation to a new training load occurs. The key is recognizing overtraining is recognizing that this performance incompetence doesn't get better with recovery / regeneration.

Of course, recognizing overtraining after it has occurred is kind of like taking the flamethrower away from your kid after the house is burning down. A smoke detector would have been helpful. Or, you know, maybe you shouldn't have given your kid the flamethrower in the first place. You get the idea.

To understand overtraining, it is important to realize where it comes from. It is intimately related to the "no pain, no gain" mentality. Athletes and coaches remember that the best performances often come after the hardest training. This leads them to continually elevate training load (by often unreasonable amounts) in a dangerous game of diminishing returns. Once the athlete goes over the edge, performance begins to decrease. The knee jerk reaction to the decreasing performance is increasing training, leading to a cycle that leads to injury and burnout. So, the first step to preventing overtraining is recognizing that the mentality of both the athlete and coach must change. Substantial increases in training load must come judiciously, and only after a plateau in performance. If the athlete is already training quite hard, and performance is continually falling, there is a problem and the answer *isn't* more training.

The next important thing to understand is that athletes respond better to variety than monotony. Some of the early (and very interesting) studies on this were performed in race horses using heart rate to quantify training load.[49] When the horses were exposed to progressively increased training volumes on an alternating "hard day / easy day" schedule, that is, the horses alternated endurance running with interval workouts, the horses adapted well to the training and increased their performance ability. However, if the trainers increased the training on the easy day, the horses rapidly developed the equivalent of overtraining. They became sluggish, irritable, and their appetites decreased, leading to weight loss.

Similar results were found in humans by Lehman et al.[50] Athletes were exposed to large increases training load through larger quantities of endurance training. This lead to poor performance and

---

The Rules of Recovery

Rule #1: Training load should only be substantially increased if there is a plateau in performance. It may be *gently* increased if performance is improving and the athlete is *clearly* not in any trouble.

Rule #2: Monotony kills. Keep easy days easy, hard days hard.

Rule #3: Athletes must rest as hard as they train.

symptoms of overtraining. Conversely, athletes athletes exposed to similar increases in intensity responded positively.

Taken together, these data would seem to indicate that overtraining can best be avoided by maintaining a clear demarcation between hard and easy days in the microcycle.

Training disturbs the homeostasis of the body. From the time you start out on a run, through the time you ran your intervals, to the time you returned home, your body went through a myriad of biochemical changes: plasma stress hormones, lactate concentration, local muscle glycogen depletion, and the like. Then, you must contend with muscle fatigue and soreness, the occasional blister or saddle sore, etc.

Your goal is to restore homeostasis as much as possible between workouts. This means learning to rest and recover as hard as you train. Although a bit extreme, the old cycling adage holds some water: Never walk when you can ride, never stand when you can sit, never sit when you can lie down. The overarching idea is that you need to control the things you can. Be sure to get enough sleep. Manage travel stress effectively by avoiding training hard on long travel days. Eat healthy and be sure you are always getting enough carbohydrates before, during, and after workouts.

CHAPTER 10
Guidelines For Racing

There are lots of people out there who are trying to set the "rules" for racing using power and pace. Some of them can get pretty esoteric. The truth is that it just doesn't need to be that complicated. (Thus, this will be a very short chapter!) However, to race to your potential, you need to be willing to do some experimenting. There is only one rule you need concern yourself with. The ABC rule. The best part about this rule is that you make it yourself.

> The ABC rule:
> Your best one hour power is: A
> Your power limit for the race in question is: B (X% of A)
> Your average power / running pace for this type of race should be: C (Y% of A)

The first step is setting the power limit (B). This is a power you should not exceed for more than a couple of minutes if you plan on running to the best of your ability. Again, these are only guidelines, but they become more crucial as the race gets longer and longer. Spending a lot of time around or above 1-hour power / CP in a race that is going to last between 2 and more than 8 hours can have catastrophic consequences. 42K is a long way to walk.

Power Limit

Event	Power Ceiling (Pro)	Power Ceiling (Amateur)
Sprint	110%	105%
Olympic	105%	100%
Half-IM	100%	95%
IM	90%	85%

The second step is finding the ESTIMATED percentage of CP / CV (C) you should be able to maintain for the event. These are simply some guidelines culled from my analysis of files / splits from professional, high level amateur and middle-of-the-pack athletes.

Average Race Power

Event	Average Power (Pro)	Average Power (Amateur)
Sprint	100%	95%
Olympic	95-98%	92-95%
Half-IM	85-87%	80-85%
IM	80%	72-78%

The third step is confirming C through race simulations. Suggested distances can be found below.

Suggested Race Simulation Distance

Event	Bike Simulation	Run Simulation
Sprint	Race Distance	Race Distance
Olympic	80% Race Distance	50% Race Distance
Half-IM	70% Race Distance	40% Race Distance
IM	50-60% Race Distance	25-30% Race Distance

A successful race simulation means riding at goal race power (or harder) and then running even splits off the bike at goal race pace. If the athlete is unable to accomplish this, it is time to re-evaluate the goal race power / run pace and decide which requires revision, or if the athlete simply does not yet have the fitness to participate in the race.

Given the practicalities of swimming, there really isn't any good way of making similar analyses and applying them in the race. Your strategy will be dictated by your perceived exertion and the behavior of your competitors. The best advice for most participants is likely to find a pair of feet going about the speed you want to be going, and tucking into a draft. This is even more critical for elite competitors who must make the first pack on the bike.

It is important to remember that racing this way isn't about being a robot. One of the most useful aspects of working with power and pace is learning how your perceived exertion correlates with the objective data coming from your power meter / GPS / stopwatch. You will come to a place where you can actually tell within a small margin of error what kind of power you are putting out, and what kind of pace you are running or swimming. When you get there, you can race with very little input from your toys and pace yourself very well. However, the toys are still important. In particular, they serve as a warning signal when your subjective feelings are falling way outside where they usually do at a particular power output. They also keep you from doing anything stupid. When someone comes by you on the bike like you are standing still, your first instinct may be to try to follow them. Because you are feeling well-tapered and strong, you may be able to keep up for 20 or 30K before you blow yourself to smithereens. A power meter keeps you from having to rely on your feelings alone. If you look down and see silly numbers, it should be a giant flashing sign that reads, "SLOW DOWN!"

Epilogue

As this book was going to press, a colleague asked me, "Do you really want to be giving away all of your secrets?" Frankly, the question misses the point. There are many coaches in the world who claim to be in possession of unique or complex training theories that are the keys to success. These people typically impress upon their followers the need for secrecy. This is purely to the advantage of the coach. The very act of controlling information fosters the popular impression that they have something worth hiding in the first place. This leads to a cult of personality, rising fees, and the blind admiration of people on the outside of the enclave.

I've had both the privilege and good fortune to work with some of the finest athletes in multi-sport, both as a performance consultant and as a sports physician. I've also had the rare opportunity of reviewing the training programs of a number world class athletes across many sports. With few exceptions, almost every truly successful training program I've seen is rooted in a scientific thought process (whether the coach and/or athlete realized it or not) and the basic principles of exercise physiology. While every coach has his or her variations on the theme, *the real secret is that there are no secrets.*

That is a tough pill to swallow for many people. When we fail to live up to our own expectations, when we are frustrated by lackluster performance or even outright failure, when we are disgusted with our own physical weakness or seeming frailty of determination, we want a solution. What's more, we want it now.

The problem is that there is no easy way. You need to remember that this is a journey of years, not weeks or even months. To demand immediate gains in the short term is to invite disillusionment, or even injury. Given this, how do we "get from here to there", so to speak?

To get the best results from yourself or from an athlete you advise, you must be willing think critically and then act rationally based on that thought process. You must remain cautious of training fads and vigilant against the pseudo-science which is continually introduced into our sport in an effort to lighten your wallet. Most of all, you must be patient. Evidence-based training isn't as fast or easy as any of the shake-and-bake methodologies you may encounter. You need to spend the time recording training and performance and analyzing what works and what doesn't. At the end of the day, however, you will be vindicated by your results. What's more, you will have a deep satisfaction in the knowledge that you engineered those results, and didn't just stumble on them through blind application of something you heard from a coach or read in a book.

Happy training, and the best of luck out there!

Works Cited

1. Coyle EF, Feltner, ME, Kautz, SA, Hamilton, MT, Montain, SJ, Baylor, AM. Physiological and biomechanical factors associated with elite endurance cycling performance. *Med Sci Sports Exerc*. 1999; 23(1):93-107.

2. Coyle EF, Coggan AR, and Hopper MK. Determinants of endurance in well-trained cyclists. *J Appl Physiol*. 1988; 64(6):2622-30.

3. Jones A and Doust J. The validity of the lactate minimum test for determnation of the maximal lactate steady state. *Med Sci Sports Exerc*. 1998; 30(8):1304-1313.

4. Sharp, Rick I. Prescribing and evaluating interval training sets in swimming: A proposed model. *J Swim Res*. 9:36-40.

5. Olbrecht et al. Relationship between swimming velocity and lactic concentration during continuous and intermittent training exercises. *Int J Sports Med*. 1985; 6(2):74-7.

6. Monod, H. and Scherrer, J. The work capacity of a synergic muscle group. *Ergonomics*. 1965; 8:329 - 338.

7. Skiba, Philip Friere. Calculation of Power Output and Training Stress In Cyclsts: The development of the BikeScore Algorithm. PhysFarm Press, 2006. Available at: http://www.physfarm.com.

8. Saunders et al. Short-term plyometric training improves running economy in highly trained middle and long distance runners. *J Strength Cond Res*. 2006. 20(4):947-54.

9. Paavolainen et al. Explosive strength training improves 5km running time by improving running economy and muscle power. *J Appl Physiol*. 1999; 86: 1527-1533.

10. Spurrs, Murphy and ML Watsford. The effect of plyometric training on distance running performance. *Eur J Appl Physiol*. 2003; 89(1):1-7.

11. Turner, Owings and JA Schwayne. Improvement in running economy after 6 weeks of plyometric training. *J Strength Cond Res*. 2003; 17(1):60-7.

12. Bosch, Frans and Ronald Klomp. *Running: Biomechanics and Exercise Physiology Applied in Practice*. Elsevier Churchill Livingstone, 2005.

13. Jones, A. The physiology of the World Record Holder for the Women's Marathon. *Inter J Sports Sci Coach*. 2006; 1(2):101-15.

14. Jones A. Running economy is negatively related to sit and reach test performance in international standard distance runners. *Int J Sports Med*. 2002; 23(1):40-3.

WORKS CITED

15 Wilson et al. Aquatic plyometrics and the freestyle flip turn. *Med Sci Sports Exerc.* 2004 36(5): 206.

16 Cossor et al. The influence of plyometric training on the freestyle tumble turn. *J Sci Med Sport.* 2006; 2(2):106-16.

17 Bastiaans JJ et al. The effects of replacing a portion of endurance training by explosive strength training on performance in trained cyclists. *Eur J Appl Physiol.* 2001; 86(1):79-84.

18 Brughelli M and Cronin J. Influence of running velocity on vertical, leg and joint stiffness: modeling and recommendations for future research. *Sports Med.* 2008; 38(8):647-57.

19 Londeree BR. Effect of training on lactate/ventilatory thresholds: a meta-analysis. *Med Sci Sports Exerc.* 1997; Jun;29(6):837-43.

20 Demarle AP et al. Whichever the initial training status, any increase in velocity at LT appears as a major factor in improved time to exhaustion at the same severe velocity after training. *Arch Physiol Biochem.* 2003; 111(2):167-176.

21 Gorostiaga et al. Uniqueness of interval and continuous training at the same maintained exercise intensity. *Eur J Appl Physiol.* 1991; 63:101-107.

22 Billat V et al. Intermittent runs at the velocity associated with maximal oxygen uptake enables subjects to remain at maximal oxygen uptake for a longer time than intense but submaximal runs. *Eur J Appl Physiol.* 2000; 81:188-196.

23 Billat V et al. Interval training at VO2max: effects on aerobic performance and overtraining markers. *Med Sci Sports Exerc.* 1999; 31(1):156-163.

24 Skiba, Philip Friere. Evaluation of a Novel Training Metric in Trained Cyclists. *Med Sci Sports Exerc.* 2007; 39(5) Supplement:S448.

25 Palmer G, Noakes TD, Hawley JA. Effects of steady state versus stochastic exercise on subsequent cycing performance. *Med Sci Sports Exerc.* 1997; 29(5) 684-687.

26 Banister EW. Modeling elite athletic performance. In: MacDougall JD, Wenger HA, Green HJ, eds. Physiological Testing of the High-Performance Athlete. Champaign, IL: Human Kinetics; 1996: 403-424.

27 Coggan AR. Making sense out of apparent chaos: Analyzing on the bike power data. In: The Science of Cycling: Transforming research into practical applications for athletes and coaches. Highlighted symposium, American College of Sports Medicine 53rd Annual Meeting. *Med Sci Sports Exerc.* 2006; 38(5):S39.

28 Coggan AR. Training and racing using a power meter: an introduction. In: USA Cycling Coaching Staff, editors. USA Cycling Level II Coaching Manual. Colorado Springs; USA Cycling; 2006. p. 119-140.

29 Skiba, Philip Friere. Quantification of Training Stress in Distance Runners. *Arch Phys Med Rehabil.* 2006; 87:29.

30 Skiba, Philip Friere. Calculation of Optimal Taper Characteristics in an Amateur Triathlete. *Med Sci Sports Exerc.* 2008; 40(5) Supplement 1:S175.

31 Skiba, Philip Friere. Calculation of Power Output and Training Stress In Swimmers: The development of the SwimScore Algorithm. PhysFarm Press, 2006. Available at: http://www.physfarm.com.

32 Skiba, Philip Friere. Calculation of Power Output and Training Stress In Cyclists: The development of the BikeScore Algorithm. PhysFarm Press, 2006. Available at: http://www.physfarm.com.

33 Skiba, Philip Friere. Calculation of Power Output and Training Stress In Runners: The development of the GOVSS Algorithm. PhysFarm Press, 2006. Available at: http://www.physfarm.com.

34 Morton RH, Fitz-Clarke JR, Banister EW. Modeling human performance in running. *J Appl Physiol*. 1990; 69:1171-1177.

35 Coyle EF, Coggan AR, and Hopper MK. Determinants of endurance in well-trained cyclists. *J Appl Physiol*. 1988; 64(6):2622-30.

36 Millet et al. Modeling the transfers of training effects on performance in elite tr athletes. *Int J Sports Med*. 2003; 23(1):55-63.

37 Fitz-Clarke JR et al. Optimizing athletic performance using influence curves. *J Appl Physiol*. 1991; 71:1151-1158.

38 Bosquet et al. Effects of tapering on performance: a meta analysis. *Med Sci Sports Exerc*. 2007; 39(8):1358-1365.

39 Bosch, Frans and Ronald Klomp. *Running: Biomechanics and Exercise Physiology Applied in Practice*. Elsevier Churchill Livingstone, 2005.

40 Verkhoshansky, Yuri. The end of "periodization" in the training of high performance sport. *Leistungssport*. 1998; 28(5). Translation available at http://www.athleticscoaching.ca.

41 Matveyev, LP. About the construction of training. *Teoriya I Praktika Fizichesckoi Kultury*. December 1991. No 12. English translation available at http://www.athleticscoaching.ca.

42 Tschiene P and Reiss M. Developmental reserves in endurance sports. *Leisstungsport*. November 1996; 25(6). Translation available at http://www.athleticscoaching.ca.

43 Verkoshansky, Y. The block training system in endurance running. Verkoshansky.com. 2007. Available at http://www.verkhoshansky.com.

44 Verkhoshansky Y, Hab D. The training system in middle distance running. *Sport Strength Training Methodology*. December 2007; No. 3. Originally published in *AthleticsStudi*, Italian Track and Field Federation. January 1999. Available at http://www.verkhoshansky.com.

45 Verkhoshansky, Y. Organization principles for training of high performance athletes. *Teoriya I Praktika Fizicheskoi Kultury*, 1991; No. 2. English translation available at http://www.verkhoshansky.com.

46 Shephard RJ. The athlete's heart: is big beautiful? *Br J Sports Med*. 1996; 30(1): 5-10.

47 Lehmann, M., P. Baumgartl, C. Wiesenack, et al. Training-overtraining: Influence of a defined increase in training volume vs training intensity on performance, catecholamines and some metabolic parameters in experienced middle and long distance runners. *Eur J Appl Physiol*. 1992; 64:169-177.

48 Foster, C. Monitoring training in athletes with reference to overtraining syndrome. *Med Sci Sports Exerc*. 1998; (30)7:1164-1168.

49 Bruin, G., H. Kuipers, H. A. Keizer, and G. J. Vandervuisse. Adaptation and overtraining in horses subjected to increasing training loads. *J Appl Physiol*. 1994. 76:1908-1913.

50 Lehmann, M., P. Baumgartl, C. Wiesenack, et al. Training-overtraining: Influence of a defined increase in training volume vs training intensity on performance, catecholamines and some metabolic parameters in experienced middle and long distance runners. *Eur J Appl Physiol*. 1992; 64:169-177.

About the Author

Dr. Philip Skiba received his medical degree in June of 2003, and trained in Physical Medicine and Rehabilitation at Georgetown University/National Rehabilitation Hospital, in Washington DC. After completing his residency in Family Medicine, he did a fellowship in Sports Medicine. He is board certified in Family Medicine, and has passed the board exams in Sports Medicine. Dr. Skiba is an attending physician at Jersey Shore Sports Medicine/Jersey Shore University Medical Center, where he treats patients and instructs the next generation of medical students, resident physicians and Sports Medicine fellows.

Dr. Skiba has been an endurance sports coach for almost 15 years, and works with amateur, elite and professional athletes around the world through his company, PhysFarm Training Systems LLC. He combines his academic, clinical and coaching background through his research work in training management and performance prediction. He regularly presents his work for the public at the major sports medicine meetings, and frequently lectures both in the U.S. and abroad on the appropriate training and health management of athletes.